Functional Anatomy for Sport and Exercise

Functional Anatomy for Sport and Exercise is a quick reference guide to human musculoskeletal anatomy in its moving, active context.

An accessible format makes it easy for students to locate clear, concise explanations and descriptions of anatomical structures, human movement terms and key concept as they are needed. Covering all major anatomical areas, the book includes:

- A simple, comprehensive guide to functional musculoskeletal anatomy
- Cross-referenced entries throughout
- Highlighting of key terms
- Hot Topics explained in more detail
- Full references and a list of suggested further reading.

Functional Anatomy for Sport and Exercise is a must-have supplement for undergraduates in applied anatomy, functional anatomy, kinesiology, physical education, strength and conditioning, biomechanics and related areas

Clare E. Milner PhD is Assistant Professor of Biomechanics in the Department of Exercise, Sport, and Leisure Studies, University of Tennessee, USA. Her teaching in the Exercise Science Program includes the Biomechanics of Orthopaedic Rehabilitation and Applied Anatomy. Her research focuses on the biomechanics of lower extremity injuries and rehabilitation, including stress fractures in runners.

D0207390

Functional Anatomy for Sport and Exercise

Quick Reference

Clare E. Milner

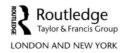

Routledge
Taylor & Francis Group

LONDON AND NEW YORK

First published 2008
by Routledge
2 Park Square, Milton Park, Abingdon, Oxon OX14 4RN

Simultaneously published in the USA and Canada
by Routledge
270 Madison Ave, New York, NY 10016

Routledge is an imprint of the Taylor & Francis Group, an informa business

© 2008 Clare E. Milner

Typeset in Sabon by
HWA Text and Data Management, London
Illustrations by Stephen Crumly
Printed and bound in Great Britain by
TJ International Ltd, Padstow, Cornwall

British Library Cataloguing in Publication Data
A catalogue record for this book is available from the British Library

Library of Congress Cataloging-in-Publication Data

Milner, Clare E.
Functional anatomy for sport and exercise : quick reference / Clare E.
Milner.
    p. ; cm.
  Includes bibliographical references and index.
  1. Musculoskeletal system—Anatomy—Handbooks, manuals, etc.
  2. Musculoskeletal system—Anatomy—Encyclopedias. 3. Sports—
Physiological aspects—Handbooks, manuals, etc. I. Title.
  [DNLM: 1. Musculoskeletal System—anatomy & histology—
Handbooks. 2. Exercise—physiology—Handbooks. WE 39 M659 2008]
  QM100.M55 2008
  612.7—dc22   2007049884

ISBN10: 0-415-43296-0 (hbk)
ISBN10: 0-415-43297-9 (pbk)

ISBN13: 978-0-415-43296-2 (hbk)
ISBN13: 978-0-415-43297-9 (pbk)

To KVJ, for your unwavering love and support

Contents

A to Z entries

Hot Topics

Figures

Acknowledgements

First and foremost, I would like to thank Samantha Grant at Routledge UK for conceiving the idea of an A to Z style musculoskeletal anatomy text for students of sport and exercise science. I am also grateful to the editors of the *Encyclopedia of International Sports Studies* for inviting me to contribute to their comprehensive text and, indirectly, introducing me to Samantha. This book would be a shadow of itself without the illustrations found throughout that add meaning and structure to the descriptions of bones and bony landmarks, my thanks to Stephen Crumly. Finally, I thank the staff at Routledge UK for their assistance at every step of the way.

Introduction

This A to Z guide is intended to provide a quick and easily accessible reference for students of musculoskeletal anatomy. It is an appropriate supplement to the traditional anatomy textbook in undergraduate courses such as applied anatomy, functional anatomy, and kinesiology. Given the applied focus of the subject matter, details of common sports and other injuries are included alongside the purely anatomical descriptions of each region. The book makes comprehensive reference information available in a concise and easily accessible format. Relevant information about musculoskeletal anatomy can be located quickly and easily without searching through a traditional anatomy textbook that includes details of all of the systems of the body. The compact format of the textbook and A to Z arrangement of entries enables topics of interest to be located quickly and easily.

Entries are grouped by major joint and include a general introduction to the region, plus detailed descriptions of the bones, joints, ligaments, and muscles. The bones of each joint are illustrated in a detailed figure including several views to ensure all of the key bony landmarks are shown. These landmarks tie in with the descriptions of ligaments and muscles and their attachments to the bone. The figure labels are lined up on the left and right sides of the diagram. This arrangement is a study tool which enables the labels to be easily covered and then revealed one by one. In this way the figures can be used to test your knowledge of the bones and their landmarks. The focus of the book is on joints that are involved in movement, including joints of the extremities, vertebral column and thoracic cage.

Key terminology and essential background information, such as the anatomical planes and axes, are also described to provide the reader with a comprehensive reference. In fact, these entries are a good place to start and will facilitate the reader's understanding of the entries describing the different regions of the body. Suggested entries for the reader who is not familiar with (or needs reminding of) the basic concepts and language of anatomy are:

Anatomical position
Anatomical terminology
Appendicular skeleton
Articular surfaces
Axial skeleton
Bone
Bony landmarks
Bone classification
Joints
Joint classification
Muscle contraction – types
Muscle classification
Planes and axes of movement

The A to Z entries are cross-referenced extensively throughout the text to guide the reader to related information about the region of interest. Further reading suggestions are also provided where appropriate. These direct the reader to both textbooks and selected research articles. In addition, there are five 'Hot Topics' boxes which provide further information about contemporary items of interest related to musculoskeletal anatomy, such as anterior cruciate ligament injuries in athletes.

A to Z entries

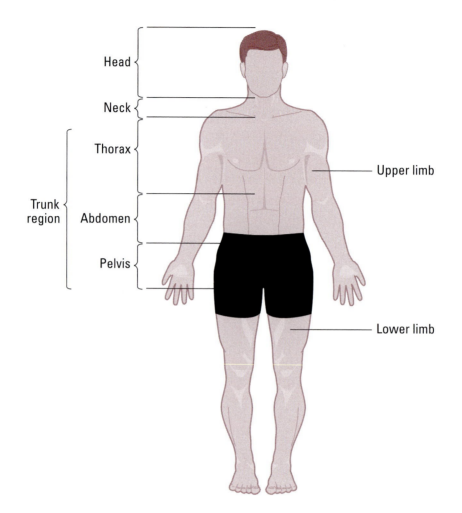

Figure 1 Anatomical position and regions of the body

Anatomical position

The anatomical position is the reference position of the body that is used when describing movements of parts of the body (Figure 1). This ensures that movement terminology is consistent, since all axes of rotation are aligned consistently throughout the upper and lower body. The position is standing upright with the head and feet pointing directly forwards, eyes looking straight ahead. The lower limbs are close together with the feet parallel. The upper limbs are down at the sides of the body with the palms of the hands facing forwards. This position of the upper limbs is different to their natural position during relaxed standing, in which the palms face the body. However, with the upper limbs in the palms-forward position, the flexion – extension axes of the elbow, wrist and joints of the hand are aligned mediolaterally. This puts them in the same orientation as the flexion – extension axes of the other joints of the body. Similarly, the abduction – adduction and internal – external rotation axes are also aligned with the rest of the body. Even though the upper limb may move to a position very different to the anatomical position, the naming of the joint rotations remains the same as in the anatomical position. When interpreting the component parts of a complex upper body movement, it can be helpful to imagine moving the limb back to the anatomical position. It will then be easier to isolate the individual joint movement and identify the axis of rotation and direction of movement.

See also **anatomical terminology; planes and axes of movement.**

Anatomical terminology

When referring to movements of the body or locations of anatomical structures in the body, specific terminology is used. The **planes and axes of movement** are used to describe movements meaningfully and unambiguously. However, the relative locations of parts of the body with respect to the whole also need to be described unambiguously.

The relative location of a point on the **axial skeleton** or **appendicular skeleton** is indicated by the use of either 'proximal' or 'distal'. A point that is more proximal lies closer to the axial skeleton than one that is more distal on the extremity. For example, the elbow lies proximal to the wrist. Similarly, a point that is more 'cranial' is closer to the head than one that is 'caudal' to it. So, the sternum (breastbone) is cranial to the pelvis. Superior and inferior are used to describe points that are above and below each other, respectively. For example, the head is superior to the neck. Whether a point is on the front or the back of the body or a segment is indicated by the use of anterior and posterior respectively, for example, the anterior and posterior heads of the deltoid muscle (*see* **shoulder complex – muscles**). 'Ventral' and 'dorsal' are alternative anatomical terms for the front and the back of the body, such that the pectoral (chest) muscles lie ventrally on the thorax and the trapezius muscle lies dorsally on the upper thorax.

To determine on which side of a segment a point lays, 'medial' is used to indicate a point that is closer to the midline of the body and 'lateral' indicates that a point is further away from the midline. For example, the medial malleolus is the bone on the inside of the ankle, closer to the midline, and the lateral malleolus is the bone on the outside of the ankle, further away from the midline (*see* **ankle and foot – bones**). Finally, to indicate how close to the center of a segment a point lies, the terms superficial and deep are used, such that skin is superficial to muscle.

See also **anatomical position; planes and axes of movement.**

Ankle and foot

The ankle and foot form a complex region containing many joints, which provide flexibility and enable the foot to adapt to its environment. This flexibility of the foot is essential because it is the point of contact between the ground and the body; it must be able to adapt to changes in terrain with minimum perturbation of the body system as a whole. The many bones and joints in the foot enable it to play multiple roles during activity; it is a flexible shock-attenuating structure during the early part of the stance phase of walking, and then becomes a rigid lever during push-off at the end of the stance phase. This change in dynamic function is achieved by activity of the invertor and evertor muscles of the foot (*see* **ankle and foot – muscles**). These rotate the foot about its longitudinal axis from a flexible pronated position to a rigid supinated position (*see* **ankle and foot – joints**).

Owing to the foot's position as the most distal segment in the body, the ankle and foot region is subjected to high loads, particularly during running and jumping activities. It is also subjected to large shear forces during cutting and other side-step activities that occur in sports. As a result of these high loads and extreme positions, the ankle and foot are at high risk of overuse injury. Additionally, injuries related to ankle and foot risk factors may manifest themselves higher up the kinetic chain – in the leg, knee, or hip. Overuse injuries related to foot and ankle structure and mechanics include plantar fasciitis, patellofemoral pain (*see* **Hot Topic 2**), tibial stress fractures (*see* **Hot Topic 1**), and chondromalacia patellae.

Further reading

Sarrafian, S.K. (1993) *Anatomy of the Foot and Ankle: Descriptive, Topographic, Functional*, Philadelphia, PA: Lippincott Williams & Wilkins.

See also **ankle and foot – bones; ankle and foot – joints; ankle and foot – ligaments; ankle and foot – muscles; appendicular skeleton; foot arches.**

Hot Topic I: tibial stress fractures in runners

Stress fractures are a common overuse injury in runners. The most common site of a stress fracture is the tibia, typically in the region about a third of the way up the bone from the ankle. Female runners are at higher risk of tibial stress fracture than male runners, although it is unclear what the cause of the difference is. A stress fracture develops when microscopic damage that is done to the bone during repeated loading accumulates over time. Bone constantly repairs itself and, in the healthy runner, the rate of repair or remodeling of the bone keeps pace with the rate of microdamage. This enables the bone to remain healthy and even become stronger over time to better withstand the repeated pavement pounding. However, if the balance is tipped and the rate of damage exceeds the rate of repair, microcracks in the bone eventually join up and a stress fracture occurs. A runner takes about 500 steps during every mile of running, each one subjecting the body to a peak force of about three times the body's weight. It is easy to appreciate the huge cumulative load experienced by the lower limbs over a period of weeks or months of running.

Numerous factors contribute to the development of a stress fracture and can tip the balance between damage and repair. Some of these can be modified to try and reduce the risk of injury. Structural factors such as the shape of the bone may predispose some runners to injury, but these cannot be altered. External factors related to training may also contribute and these can be altered to reduce the risk of injury. For example, the running surface and shoe used should provide some cushioning and shock absorption to reduce the load on the limb. Therefore, running on grass in cushioned running shoes is preferable to running on concrete in stiff-soled shoes. The training program may also be a cause of injury. Increasing the weekly mileage (the total load on the body) too quickly can tip the balance and cause the bone to be damaged more quickly than it can be repaired. Poor nutrition can also weaken the bone and reduce bone density, lowering the threshold at which damage will exceed the rate of repair. This is a special concern among competitive distance runners who diet to reduce their body weight as much as possible and restrict their intake of essential nutrients. The biomechanics of running (running technique) may also be an important factor. For example, some runners tend to hit the ground harder with every step, even after differences in weight are taken into consideration. These runners will have a higher total load on the body for every mile of running compared to those who are lighter on their feet.

After a tibial stress fracture, a period of rest and rehabilitation of up to 12 weeks is needed to allow the bone to remodel and repair itself. After sustaining a stress fracture once, the runner is quite likely to get the same injury in the future if they keep doing the same things they were before the injury. To avoid another stress fracture, special attention should be paid to factors such as the training program, nutrition, and running biomechanics to correct any deficiencies which may put the athlete at increased risk of injury.

After fracture healing, several measures are available to try and prevent recurrence of the stress fracture. The most easily manipulated risk factor is training load and frequency; individuals should restart their training programmes conservatively and be cautious about increasing either the length or intensity of individual sessions, or the number of sessions. Similarly, softer training surfaces can be chosen and appropriate footwear with adequate shock absorption capabilities and support should be worn. Other options include orthotics (*see* **Hot Topic 2**), which are fitted into the running shoe to realign the position of the foot, if faulty mechanics are suspected. Gait retraining is an option that is being developed and applied to reduce the risk of overuse injuries in at-risk runners.

Further reading

Bennell, K. and Brukner, P. (2005) 'Preventing and managing stress fractures in athletes', *Physical Therapy in Sport*, 6: 171–80.

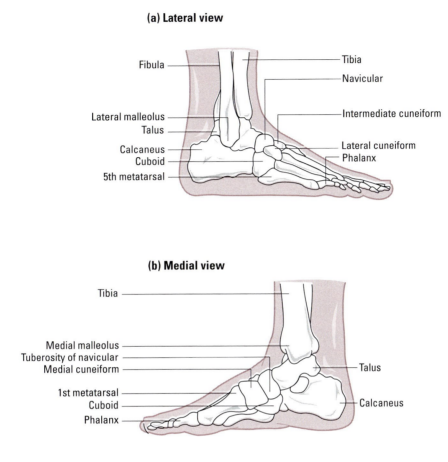

(a) Lateral view

Fibula

Tibia

Navicular

Intermediate cuneiform

Lateral malleolus

Talus

Calcaneus

Cuboid

5th metatarsal

Lateral cuneiform

Phalanx

(b) Medial view

Tibia

Medial malleolus

Tuberosity of navicular

Medial cuneiform

1st metatarsal

Cuboid

Phalanx

Talus

Calcaneus

Figure 2 Bones of the right foot and ankle

Ankle and foot – bones

The ankle and foot contain many bones and joints, giving the region high mobility. As the first point of contact between the body and the ground, this flexible segment enables the individual to adapt easily to changes in terrain. The bones of the ankle joint are those of the distal part of the leg – the tibia and fibula – and the talus. The twenty-six bones of the foot are the talus, calcaneus, navicular, cuboid, and the three cuneiforms – these are the tarsal bones – plus the five metatarsal bones and the fourteen phalanges (Figure 2).

The talus is common to both the ankle and the foot, forming the distal part of the ankle joint and the proximal part of the subtalar joint. The distal ends of the tibia and fibula, the malleoli, form the proximal part of the ankle joint and can be used to approximate the ankle joint axis *in vivo*. The ankle joint axis passes just distal to the tips of the malleoli; according to Inman (1976) the axis lies, on average, 5 mm distal to the tip of the medial malleolus, and 3 mm distal and 8 mm anterior to the tip of the lateral malleolus.

The bones of the foot and ankle are at risk of stress fracture, particularly in runners and military recruits. Stress fractures commonly occur in the navicular, the metatarsals and the distal third of the tibia. There is some evidence that the incidence of these overuse injuries is higher in those individuals who have narrower tibiae, since these bones are less able to resist the bending forces to which the leg is subjected when the foot contacts the ground on every stride. Furthermore, stress fractures occur twice as often in females than in males, although the reasons for this difference are unclear. Owing to the seriousness of stress fractures, which require several weeks rest from training and physical activity until the bone is healed, they are an important research topic for sports biomechanists and physical therapists. Factors that are thought to be related to the risk of stress fracture include structural anatomy, functional mechanics, footwear and training surface, training load, training frequency, and sex (*see* **Hot Topic 1**).

See also ankle and foot; ankle and foot – joints; ankle and foot – ligaments; ankle and foot – muscles; foot arches.

Ankle and foot – joints

The ankle and foot form a complex of many joints that provides flexibility and enables the foot to adapt to its environment. This flexibility of the foot is essential because it is the point of contact between the ground and the body; it must be able to adapt to changes in terrain with minimum perturbation of the body system as a whole. The foot is often divided into three sections based on its major articulations. The rear foot consists of the ankle and subtalar joints, the midfoot contains the calcaneocuboid, cuneonavicular, cuboideonavicular, intercuneiform, and cuneocuboid joints, and the forefoot consists of the tarsometatarsal, intermetatarsal, metatarsophalangeal, and interphalangeal joints. The greatest range of foot and ankle motion occurs at the rear foot.

The ankle, or talocrural, joint is the link between the leg and the foot. It approximates a hinge joint, with the talus of the foot being surrounded by the lateral malleolus, the medial malleolus, and the distal end of the tibia. Sagittal plane flexion – extension movements at the ankle are known as plantarflexion, pointing the toes away from the leg, and dorsiflexion, pulling the toes towards the leg. From the neutral position, with the foot at 90° to the leg, the ankle can move into about 20° of dorsiflexion and 50° of plantarflexion.

The subtalar, or talocalcaneal, joint is formed between the distal surface of the talus and the proximal surface of the calcaneus. The subtalar joint axis is oriented obliquely in an anteromedial and superior direction. Since the joint axis is not aligned with any of the three cardinal planes of the body, movements about it are described as triplanar, with rotations occurring about all three anatomical axes. Movement about the subtalar joint axis is described as pronation, in which the rear foot rolls inwards towards its medial side, or supination, in which the rear foot rolls in the opposite direction. Rear foot pronation consists of eversion, dorsiflexion, and external rotation; its converse, supination, is made up of inversion, plantarflexion, and internal rotation.

The subtalar joint plays an important role in the shock absorption mechanism of the foot, owing to the changing properties of the foot as it moves from the rigid supinated position to the flexible pronated position. Abnormalities of rear foot motion have been associated with overuse injuries that can occur during running. During walking and running, the rotation of the rear foot about the subtalar joint axis helps to attenuate the forces transmitted through the foot and into the contact limb at foot strike. In a normal gait cycle, the foot contacts the ground in a supinated position, with the posterolateral part of the heel contacting first. The foot then moves into pronation, reaching a maximum towards the middle of the stance phase when the foot is flat on the ground. Finally, the foot returns to supination at toe off. The large rotation movement at foot strike, from supination to maximum pronation, is a shock-absorbing mechanism. The rate of pronation of the rear foot of the support limb at foot strike has been implicated in injury risk. Similarly, the maximum pronation reached during midstance is also thought to be linked to overuse injuries of the lower extremities, such as patellofemoral pain and Achilles tendon injury. The foot returns to supination towards toe off to provide a rigid lever during the push off at the end of stance phase. Failure of the foot to return to its rigid configuration has also been linked with overuse injury.

The joints of the midfoot have a much smaller range of motion than those of the rear foot and function mainly by gliding and rotating, providing a link between the independently articulating rear foot and forefoot regions.

The relationship between the rear foot and the forefoot articulations is generally one of opposite rotation, which enables the sole of the foot to remain flat on the ground during complex movements such as sidestep cutting. Forefoot inversion – eversion occurs mainly at the transverse tarsal joint. This 'joint' is made up of the five tarsometatarsal joints, which are the proximal articulations of the metatarsal bones. During a sidestep cut, the drive leg is at an oblique angle to the ground in the frontal plane. Consequently, the rear foot must be supinated to enable the heel to remain flat on the ground. If the foot was not a flexible, multi-articulated segment, this would result in the forefoot having minimal contact on its medial border and being overloaded on its lateral border. Because of the multi-joint configuration of the foot, the forefoot rotates in the opposite direction to the rotation of the rear foot, into forefoot eversion, enabling weight to be distributed evenly over the whole of the sole of the foot.

The metatarsophalangeal joints at the base of the toes also play an important role during locomotion and have a large range of flexion – extension motion. Active extension in these joints, curling the toes up towards the ankle, from the neutral position, is typically 50° to 60°, much greater than the 30° or 40° of flexion that can be achieved from that position; this is an adaptation to the role of the foot during walking. During toe off at the end of the stance phase of gait, the ankle is plantarflexed and the foot is supinated to provide a rigid lever to push off from the ground. The large extension possible at the metatarsophalangeal joints enables more of the toe region to remain in contact with the ground as the ankle plantarflexes and points the foot during this push off phase. This provides a larger base of support during the terminal stance phase.

Further reading

Whittle, M.W. (2001) *Gait Analysis: An Introduction*, Oxford: Butterworth Heinemann.

See also **ankle and foot; ankle and foot – bones; ankle and foot – ligaments; ankle and foot – muscles; gait analysis.**

Ankle and foot – ligaments

The ankle and foot contain many small bones and these are held together by ligaments. The ligaments of the ankle are grouped into lateral and medial collateral ligaments. The ankle ligaments are named according to the bones that they join together. Key bones are the leg bones the tibia and fibula, which form the proximal part of the ankle joint, and the foot bones the talus and the calcaneus. The lateral collateral ligament complex consists of the anterior talofibular ligament, the calcaneofibular ligament, and the posterior talofibular ligament. The three ligaments are thin bands of tissue and are relatively weak and susceptible to injury. The lateral ankle ligaments are the most commonly damaged ligaments in the body. The mechanism of injury is to 'roll' or 'sprain' your ankle, the common description of an inversion injury. When you sprain your ankle in this way, the anterior ligament is torn first, followed by the calcaneofibular and then the posterior ligament, as the severity of the injury increases. If the ligaments do not heal correctly, either remaining incomplete or becoming longer than before the injury, the ankle will be mechanically unstable and at greater risk of further injury to the lateral ligament. Following ligament damage, joint proprioception is typically reduced, which is also a factor in the predisposition of the individual for future recurrence of the injury.

The medial collateral ligament of the ankle is also known as the deltoid ligament. It is so called because it is triangular in shape. The deltoid ligament is thick and strong and not divided into discrete bands like the lateral collateral ligaments. However, the medial ligaments of the ankle can also be identified according to the bones that they hold together. The names of the individual components vary slightly depending on which textbook you read, precisely because they are not conveniently separated like the lateral ligaments. The following is a common nomenclature for the components of the deltoid ligament. From anterior to posterior: tibionavicular (part of this ligament also attaches to the talus, referred to as anterior tibiotalar), tibiocalcaneal, and posterior tibiotalar. Since the deltoid ligament is thick and strong, it is not commonly injured. However, the mechanism of injury is the opposite movement to the mechanism of injury of the lateral collateral ligaments: an eversion sprain.

In addition to the medial and lateral collateral ligaments, there are two other ligaments at the distal end of the tibia and fibula. These are the anterior and posterior tibiofibular ligaments. These short ligaments bind the distal end of the tibia and fibular together tightly, to minimize any movement between them. The distal tibiofibular joint can effectively be considered to be immovable, with nothing more than a small amount of 'give' possible between the two leg bones.

There are many ligaments in the foot, too many to name individually. Their main function is to maintain the integrity of the foot system, which consists of 26 different bones. Since the foot has to function both as a flexible shock absorber during contact with the ground and a rigid lever while pushing off from the ground, the ligaments must allow some movement between adjacent bones, but not a large amount. The shape of the bones of the foot and the way that they fit together also provides a large amount of stability in the foot, as do the intrinsic and extrinsic foot muscles. Finally, another soft tissue structure, the plantar aponeurosis, runs along the sole of the foot and provides additional support for the **foot arches**.

See also **ankle and foot; ankle and foot – bones; ankle and foot – joints; ankle and foot – muscles; foot arches.**

Ankle and foot – muscles

The ankle and foot form a complex structure containing many bones and joints, which provide flexibility and enable the foot to adapt to its environment. This flexibility is essential because the foot is the first point of contact between the ground and the body and must be able to adapt to changes in terrain with minimum perturbation of the body as a whole. The muscles of the foot and ankle enable this flexible structure to perform different roles. For example, during walking and running the foot acts as both a shock absorber and a rigid lever at different points in the gait cycle.

The muscles of the ankle and foot can be divided into four groups: the anterior leg muscles, the posterior leg (calf) muscles, the lateral leg muscles, and the intrinsic muscles of the foot. The anterior muscles are the tibialis anterior, peroneus tertius, extensor digitorum longus, and extensor hallucis longus. As a group, these muscles are responsible for dorsiflexion of the ankle. In addition, tibialis anterior supinates the foot, peroneus tertius pronates the foot, extensor digitorum longus extends the four lesser toes and pronates the foot, and extensor hallucis longus supinates the foot and extends the big toe.

The posterior muscles of the ankle and foot are gastrocnemius, soleus, plantaris, flexor digitorum longus, flexor hallucis longus, and tibialis posterior. As a group, these muscles are responsible for plantarflexion of the ankle. Gastrocnemius is the large two-headed muscle that forms the bulk of the calf and is also a flexor of the knee (*see* **knee – muscles**). The next largest muscle of the calf is soleus, which lies deep to the gastrocnemius; its action is purely ankle plantarflexion. Between these two muscles lies the small plantaris muscle, which makes a minor contribution to knee flexion and plantarflexion. Deep to these muscles lies popliteus; this muscle contributes to knee flexion and internal rotation of the tibia. Flexors digitorum and hallucis longus perform the opposite function to the extensor muscle groups on the anterior aspect of the leg. Tibialis posterior supinates the foot in addition to plantarflexing the ankle. Two muscles are situated laterally on the leg: peroneus longus and peroneus brevis. Their role is pronation and plantarflexion. The intrinsic muscles of the foot contribute to movement of the toes. There are many muscles within the foot, with the muscles of the dorsum of the foot being four layers deep.

See also **ankle and foot; ankle and foot – bones; ankle and foot – joints; ankle and foot – ligaments; foot arches; gait analysis.**

Appendicular skeleton

The appendicular skeleton consists of the bones of the upper and lower limbs and the shoulder and pelvic girdles, through which the limbs attach to the axial skeleton (Figure 3). The upper limb can be divided into the arm, forearm, and hand. Similarly, the lower limb can be divided into the thigh, leg, and foot.

The upper limb bones are the humerus in the arm, the ulna and radius in the forearm, and the carpals, metacarpals, and phalanges of the hand. The shoulder girdle consists of the clavicles (collarbones), which attach to the sternum (breastbone) medially, and the scapulae (shoulder blades), which are connected to the trunk by muscular attachments only. The major joints of the upper limb are the shoulder, elbow, wrist, and the articulations of the individual digits.

The shoulder is a ball and socket joint. The ball is the proximal end of the humerus, which sits in the shallow socket of the scapula known as the glenoid fossa (*see* **shoulder complex – joints**). This enables the shoulder to be extremely versatile in its movements and it is capable of multiaxial rotation (*see* **planes and axes of movement**). The humerus is held in place by strong ligaments and tendinous attachments. The elbow is a hinge joint formed by the articulation of the humerus and ulna and, therefore, has one main axis of rotation, for flexion – extension (*see* **elbow – joints**). The articulation between the radius and the ulna is responsible for pronation and supination of the hand. With the elbow flexed to 90° from the anatomical position, the hand is in a supinated position when it is palm up and pronated when palm down. This movement is achieved by the radius crossing over the ulna in the forearm. The wrist lies between the ulna and radius of the forearm and the metacarpal bones of the hand. This joint is biaxial, permitting flexion – extension and abduction-adduction (*see* **wrist and hand – joints**).

The lower limb bones are the femur in the thigh, the patella (kneecap), the tibia (shin bone) and fibula in the calf, and the tarsals, metatarsals, and phalanges in the foot. The pelvic girdle is made up of the hip bones, the os coxae, each of which comprises the ilium, ischium, and pubis. The pelvis is a much more rigid structure than the light and mobile shoulder girdle. The major joints of the lower limb are the hip, knee, ankle, subtalar joint, and the joints of the foot.

There are some similarities between the upper and lower limbs. The hip joint is a ball and socket joint, like the shoulder, but the femur is set more deeply into the hip bone. Comparable to the shoulder, the hip is capable of multiaxial rotation and is the most mobile joint of the lower extremity. When bearing weight, the knee is primarily a hinge joint, like the elbow; its major movement is flexion – extension. Only the larger bone of the leg, the tibia, contributes to the knee joint. Both the tibia and fibula contribute to the ankle, along with the talus. The ankle is also a hinge joint: rotation of the foot about the other two axes of rotation is achieved through the oblique subtalar joint of the rear foot.

See also **axial skeleton; ankle and foot – bones; elbow and forearm – bones; hip – bones; knee – bones; shoulder complex – bones; wrist and hand – bones.**

AXIAL   **APPENDICULAR**

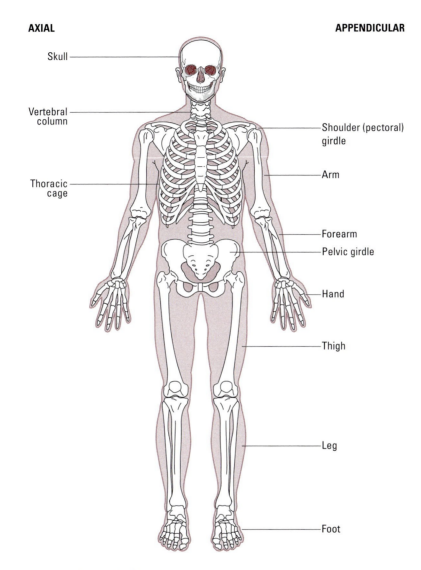

Skull

Vertebral
column

Thoracic
cage

Shoulder (pectoral)
girdle

Arm

Forearm

Pelvic girdle

Hand

Thigh

Leg

Foot

Figure 3 Axial and appendicular skeleton

Articulating surfaces

Articulating surfaces are the cartilage-covered ends of bone which touch adjacent bones at joints. In synovial joints, these surfaces are covered with articular hyaline cartilage. Hyaline cartilage is flexible and resilient, providing a cushion between the ends of the bones where they come into contact with each other. The cartilage is able to absorb some of the compressive forces at the joint, and so help to protect the bone from damage. Cartilage itself does not contain any blood vessels or nerves. This means that it relies on the fluid which surrounds it (synovial fluid) for nutrients. The compressive forces that occur at the joint as it is loaded help to move these fluids into and out of the cartilage. This happens in a similar way to squeezing a sponge which is submerged in a bowl of water: as the sponge is squeezed, water is forced out, then when the pressure is released water rushes back into the sponge. This is why it is important to load the joints regularly to keep them healthy.

The primary function of cartilage is to protect the bone from damage by distributing the load over a large surface area, which decreases the stress at any one part of the bone's surface. Articular cartilage also helps to minimize friction between adjacent bones during movement by providing a smooth surface. These two functions of cartilage help to minimize wear and damage to the articular surfaces of the joint. This is an important role because wear and damage to the articulating surfaces is a precursor to the development of osteoarthritis at the joint. This is a painful condition in which the protective cartilage is damaged and wears away, leaving the bones directly in contact with one another. Osteoarthritis is a major cause of reduced mobility in older adults, primarily affecting the knees and hips, which are the major weight-bearing joints in the lower extremities.

See also **ankle and foot – joints; elbow and forearm – joints; head and neck – joints; hip – joint; joint classification; joints; knee – joints;**

lumbar spine and pelvis – joints; shoulder complex – joints; thoracic region – joints; wrist and hand – joints.

Axial skeleton

The axial skeleton consists of the vertebral column and skull plus the ribs and associated bones of the thorax (Figure 3). It is the central part of the skeleton and the **appendicular skeleton** attaches to it through the shoulder and pelvic girdles. The vertebral column contains thirty-three vertebrae in four regions; moving distally from the head, these are the seven cervical, twelve thoracic, five lumbar, five sacral, and four coccygeal vertebrae. Vertebrae within a region are numbered in ascending order in a proximal to distal direction. The sacrum and coccyx are made up of fused vertebrae, whereas the vertebrae in the other regions are movable. The vertebral column is not simply a stack of vertebrae, but has four curved regions: the cervical curve is convex anteriorly, followed by the thoracic curve, which is concave anteriorly, the anteriorly convex lumbar curve, and the anteriorly concave pelvic curve. Since the vertebrae protect the spinal cord, injuries to this region are potentially very severe. Depending on the vertebral level at which the spinal cord is damaged, more or less of the body may be paralyzed. As a result, most sports have rules that are designed to minimize the risk of spinal cord damage. For example, American football has banned tackles made with the head of the tackler as the first point of contact with the opponent. This rule was introduced after changes to protective headgear led to a large increase in cervical spine injuries following an increase in the use of this tackling technique.

The bones of the thorax (chest) form a protective cage around the major organs of the chest cavity, principally the lungs and heart. Each vertebra of the thoracic region has a pair of ribs associated with it. Of the twelve pairs of ribs, ten are attached to the sternum (breastbone) anteriorly by costal cartilage. The first seven pairs are true ribs attaching directly to the sternum via their own costal cartilage. The next three pairs are the false ribs: they attach to the sternum indirectly via the costal cartilage of the ribs above. The most distal two pairs of ribs are not secured anteriorly and are, therefore, known as floating, or free, ribs. As the link between the upper and lower body, the bones of the thorax can be subjected to large forces in those sports that call for power to be transferred from one part of the body to another. For example, rib stress fractures are relatively common in rowers. During the rowing stroke, a rower must drive his or her legs against the foot plate of the boat and subsequently transfer the power generated at the feet to the oar handle and propel the boat through the water. For the force developed at the foot plate to be transferred effectively to the blade, the trunk must provide a rigid link between the lower and upper body. The muscular tension necessary to achieve this places great strain on the ribs and may result in a stress fracture. This injury tends to occur during winter training when the rower is training at a lower stroke rate but generating more force with each stroke.

The skull consists of the cranium, the large dome that houses and protects the brain, and the bones of the face. It is made up of eight cranial and fourteen facial bones. All of these, except the mandible or jawbone, are attached rigidly to each other in the adult by interlaced articulations called sutures (*see* **joint classification**). Injuries to the skull tend to be acute trauma from contact with another athlete, equipment, or the ground.

Further reading

Warden, S.J. *et al.* (2002) 'Aetiology of rib stress fractures in rowers', *Sports Medicine*, 32: 819–36.

See also **appendicular skeleton; head and neck – bones; lumbar spine and pelvis – bones; thoracic region – bones; vertebral structure.**

Bone

Bone is hard, strong and stiff and its function is to support the soft tissues of the body and protect vital organs. It also serves as a storage site for minerals, especially calcium, and is the source of new blood cells. Bone contains calcium carbonate, calcium phosphate, collagen (a flexible fibrous protein), and water. Bone is a living tissue with living cells and it is constantly being remodeled in response to the current stresses and strains that are being applied to it.

There are two types of bone, which are classified by their porosity. The greater the volume of mineralized (calcified) tissue in the bone, the less porous it is. Cortical or compact bone has more than 70 per cent mineralized tissue by volume. This type of bone is the outside layer of bone. The bone type on the inside of a bone is more porous and is called trabecular or cancellous or spongy bone. Spongy is also a good way to describe its structure. The mineralized bone tissue forms a honeycomb structure with lots of pockets or spaces in it. The structure of trabecular bone makes bones more lightweight. The pattern of the mineralized part of the trabecular bone develops in response to the stress patterns that the bone is subjected to, with more tissue laid down in areas of high stress. This allows bone to be both light and strong. Cortical bone has a dense, solid appearance due to the high content of mineralized bone tissue, however it is not made up completely of solid mineralized tissue. Cortical bone also contains cells which lay down the mineralized tissue as well as channels for blood and lymph vessels. It should be noted that the whole of the inside of long bones is not filled with trabecular bone. The central medullary cavity down the shaft, or diaphysis, of a long bone is filled with bone marrow. This is the site of new blood cell production. Trabecular bone is only laid down at the expanded ends of long bones (the epiphyses), where it adds strength to the bone's structure in areas of high stress.

See also ankle and foot – bones; appendicular skeleton; articulating surfaces; axial skeleton; bone classification; bony landmarks; elbow and forearm – bones; head and neck – bones; hip – bones; knee – bones; lumbar spine and pelvis – bones; shoulder complex – bones; thoracic region – bones.

Bone classification

Bones can be classified according to their structure and shape. There are five categories of bone when classified by structure: long bones, short bones, flat bones, sesamoid bones and irregular bones. Long bones are those which are basically tubular: they have a long shaft. A good example is the femur in the thigh (*see* **thigh – bones**). However, the classification does not refer to the actual length of the bones; a long bone is simply longer than it is wide, like a narrow tube. The phalanges, metacarpals, and metatarsals in the hands (*see* **wrist and hand – bones**) and feet (*see* **ankle and foot – bones**) are also long bones, even though they are quite small. Short bones are those with a cuboidal shape, with width about equal to length. The tarsal and carpal bones in the feet and wrists are short bones. Flat bones are thin and flattened and typically play a protective role. They are usually curved surfaces, not flat as the name suggests. The bones of the skull (*see* **head and neck – bones**) and pelvis (*see* **lumbar spine and pelvis**) are flat bones, as well as the ribs, scapula and sternum (*see* **thoracic region – bones**). Sesamoid bones are a special category of bones that are embedded within a tendon. They are sometimes considered to be a subcategory of short bones. The best example of a sesamoid bone is the patella (kneecap), which lies within the tendon of the quadriceps muscle at the knee (*see* **knee – bones**). The patella keeps the tendon further away from the joint, which changes the angle of the tendon and enables the quadriceps muscle to produce more torque to move the joint. The pisiform in the wrist is also a sesamoid bone. There are two small sesamoid bones under the first metatarsal head in the foot, which help to protect the tendons from damage when the foot is on the ground. Sesamoid bones vary in size and shape between people and an individual may have other sesamoid bones in addition to those described. The final category is irregular bones. Irregular bones are those which do not fit into any of the other categories! The vertebrae of the spine are irregular bones (*see* **vertebral structure**).

See also ankle and foot – bones; appendicular skeleton; articulating surfaces; axial skeleton; bone; bony landmarks; elbow and forearm – bones; head and neck – bones; hip – bones; knee – bones; lumbar spine and pelvis – bones; shoulder complex – bones; thoracic region – bones.

Bony landmarks

Bones have many different landmarks at the joints and for the attachment of ligaments, tendons and muscles. Bony landmarks can be divided into articulating and non-articulating surfaces. **Articulating surfaces** are smooth cartilage-covered parts of bone that are part of the joints. Non-articulating surfaces are located at various sites on the bone where muscles and ligaments attach. A head is an articulating surface that is rounded like a ball. The head of the humerus and the head of the femur are part of ball and socket joints at the shoulder (*see* **shoulder complex – bones**) and hip (*see* **hip – bones**) respectively. A condyle is a large articulating knob that is part of a compound joint. Examples are the femoral condyles at the knee (*see* **knee – bones**). A facet is a flat or shallow articular surface found at a gliding or sliding joint (*see* **joint classification**). The facets of the superior and inferior articular processes of the vertebrae are good examples (*see* **vertebral structure**).

Non-articulating surfaces for the attachment of ligaments and tendons include large rough processes called tuberosities, such as the tibial tuberosity for the attachment of the tendon of quadriceps (*see* **knee – bones**). A small rounded process is known as a tubercle, such as the greater and lesser tubercles of the proximal humerus (*see* **shoulder complex – bones**). A process is a bony prominence, like the xiphoid process on the distal end of the sternum (*see* **thoracic region – bones**). A spine is a sharp process, such as the anterior superior iliac spine of the pelvis (*see* **lumbar spine and pelvis – bones**). An epicondyle is a projection above a condyle, such as the lateral and medial epicondyles of the femur (*see* **knee – bones**). There are two kinds of depression found on the bones: a shallow depression called a fossa and a small pit called a fovea. Examples are the iliac fossa of the pelvis (*see* **lumbar spine and pelvis – bones**) and the fovea capitis of the head of the femur (*see* **hip – bones**). There are various holes through the bones, known as foramina. For example every vertebra has a vertebral foramen for the spinal cord to pass through (*see* **vertebral structure**).

See also **anatomical terminology; appendicular skeleton; axial skeleton; bone.**

Core stability

The core region of the body is the lumbopelvic – hip complex. This includes the lumbar vertebrae, pelvis, hip joints, and the ligaments and muscles that produce or restrict movement of these segments. Stability is the ability to limit displacement and maintain structural integrity. Core stability, therefore, is the ability of the lumbopelvic – hip complex to prevent buckling of the vertebral column and return it to equilibrium following perturbation (Willson *et al.*, 2005). This area has become the focus of attention in injury prevention and rehabilitation strategies. The main concept of core stability is that the trunk (*see* **axial skeleton – structure and function**) must be stable if the extremities that are attached to it (*see* **appendicular skeleton**) are to be used safely and effectively. It relies mostly on muscular activity to increase trunk and hip stiffness.

If the core region is not stabilized effectively, excessive movement of the pelvis and lumbar spine may occur during activity. If this happens during demanding and repeated sports movements, the lower back is put under increased strain and overuse injuries resulting in lower back pain can occur. A strong and stable core is essential in most sporting activities. The role of the trunk is obvious in power transfer in sports such as rowing, during which power generated in the lower limbs must be transferred through the body to the upper limbs. However, a stable core is also important in sports without an obvious transfer of power through the torso, such as running. The role of the core muscles in running is to stabilize the pelvis as the body is supported alternately on each leg during the running stride. This is important in enabling the lower extremity to be in correct alignment when it is loaded during ground contact, an important factor in overuse injury prevention. This function of the core muscles is also important in team sports that involve rapid cutting movements and changes in direction.

The multiple muscles involved in stabilizing the core are in several layers around the abdomen (*see* **lumbar spine and pelvis – muscles**). The muscle fibers in each layer (*see* **muscles**) have a different orientation than the other layers. This arrangement provides greater stability at the core than if all the fibers were in the same direction in each layer. The same concept gives a thin sheet of multi-layered plywood its great strength. Core stability develops from the co-contraction of agonist – antagonist muscle groups (*see* **muscle contraction – types**) in each of the three planes of movement (*see* **planes and axes of movement**):

- in the sagittal plane: rectus abdominis, transverse abdominis, erector spinae, multifidus, gluteus maximus, and the hamstrings;
- in the frontal plane: gluteus medius, gluteus minimus, quadratus lumborum, adductor magnus, adductor longus, adductor brevis, and pectineus;
- in the transverse plane: gluteus maximus, gluteus medius, piriformis, superior and inferior gemelli, quadratus femoris, obturator externus and internus, internal and external obliques, iliocostalis lumborum, and multifidus.

Athletes often mistakenly focus on strengthening the surface muscle of the abdomen – rectus abdominis – in an attempt to stabilize this region. This sheet of muscle runs proximal to distal along the torso and is involved in trunk flexion; it does not provide the deep circumferential support of the lower torso for which the core muscles are responsible.

In athletes with a weak core, the core muscles may not be automatically activated to provide trunk stabilization when needed. The athlete must be trained to activate the muscles consciously during the preparatory stage of a movement to protect and stabilize the lower back. With practice, the core muscles will start to activate whenever the body is loaded and a strong core is needed.

While learning to activate the correct muscles, the athlete should sit or lie with the pelvis in a neutral position and think about drawing the navel up and in towards the spine. This is a subtle movement and, therefore, may require a different sort of body awareness than the power athlete is used to. Although the movement is small, it has a significant effect on the stability of the whole body. Another way to determine whether the transverse abdominis is being activated is to locate the place on the front of the pelvis where the muscle can be felt at the surface. On the front of the pelvis are two bony protuberances, the anterior superior iliac spines (*see* **lumbar spine and pelvis – bones**) that can be felt anteriorly just below the top of the iliac crests laterally on the pelvis. Just medial to these bony protuberances is the soft tissue region where the transverse abdominis can be felt. To learn how this muscle feels when activated, an individual should cough with their fingertips against this region – he or she should feel the muscle tighten and relax. When the transverse abdominis is consciously contracted, the same tension should be felt under the fingertips. This is a good test to use during core stability training to determine whether the correct muscles are being activated.

Further reading

Willson, J.D. *et al.* (2005) 'Core stability and its relationship to lower extremity function and injury', *Journal of the American Academy of Orthopaedic Surgeons*, 13: 316–25.

See also **lumbar spine and pelvis.**

Elbow and forearm

The elbow joint complex consists of a hinge joint between the humerus of the arm and the ulna of the forearm, plus a secondary hinge joint between the radius of the forearm and the humerus, both of which are constrained to uniaxial flexion – extension motion (*see* **planes and axes of movement**). A third joint occurs between the bones of the forearm: the proximal radioulnar joint, which is often considered to be part of the elbow joint because it is contained within the same articular capsule. The radioulnar joint allows pronation – supination of the forearm, which enables the hand to assume a pronated or supinated position at any elbow flexion angle.

In sports that have a large involvement of the upper extremity, the elbow is at risk of overuse injury. Large forces can be transmitted across the joint in hitting sports such as tennis and baseball. Overuse injuries can range from the severity of stress fractures of the humerus to tissue inflammation at tendon insertions caused by overuse of the muscle involved. These injuries are often related to incorrect technique. The many degrees of freedom of the upper extremity mean that a given movement of the hand can be achieved by many different positions and orientations of the proximal segments of the limb. Poor technique overstresses certain tissues and, as a result of the repetition of practice and competition, relatively minor deviations from the correct structural alignment of the limb can result in cumulative damage leading to overuse injury.

See also **appendicular skeleton; elbow and forearm – bones; elbow and forearm – joints; elbow and forearm – ligaments; elbow and forearm – muscles.**

Elbow and forearm – bones

The ulnohumeral joint is a hinge joint between the trochlea of the humerus in the arm and the trochlear notch of the ulna in the forearm of the upper extremity; its motion is sagittal plane flexion – extension (*see* **planes and axes of movement**). The entire joint comprises three articulations between the three long bones of the upper limb (Figure 4). These are the ulnohumeral joint already described, the radiohumeral joint between the head of the radius of the forearm and the capitulum of the humerus, and the proximal radiohumeral joint. The head of the radius is constrained by the anular ligament at the proximal radioulnar joint. This joint enables pronation and supination of the forearm. Stabilization of the elbow is provided by both the bony structure of the ulnohumeral joint, with the trochlear sitting in the trochlear notch, and by the soft tissue structures. Important soft tissue stabilizers are the joint capsule, the medial and lateral collateral ligaments, and the anular ligament that maintains the position of the proximal end of the radius at the elbow.

Traumatic injuries to the forearm are relatively common in team sports such as soccer. A player may fall and land awkwardly, with the arm extended to cushion the impact of the fall. Such a fall can result in fracture of the forearm or dislocation of the shoulder joint (*see* **shoulder complex – joints**).

See also **elbow and forearm; elbow and forearm – joints; elbow and forearm – ligaments; elbow and forearm – muscles.**

Elbow and forearm – joints

The elbow consists of three joints all within the same joint capsule. The major articulation of the elbow is the hinge joint between the humerus of the upper arm and the ulna of the forearm. This ulnohumeral joint is responsible for flexion – extension of the elbow joint. Mediolateral movement at the joint is prevented by its bony structure (*see* **planes and axes of movement**). The distal end of the humerus, the trochlea, sits in the trochlear notch at the proximal end of the ulna. The second joint at the elbow is between the radius of the forearm and the humerus. This radiohumeral joint is not constrained by its bony structure. It

(a) Anterior view

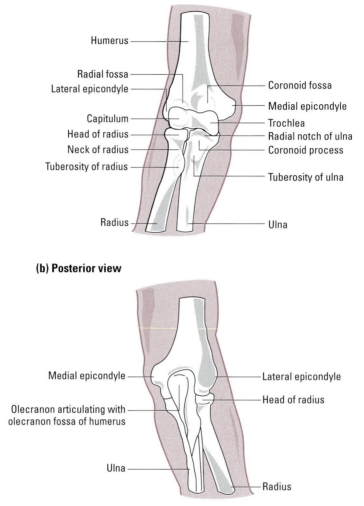

Humerus

Radial fossa

Lateral epicondyle

Capitulum

Head of radius

Neck of radius

Tuberosity of radius

Coronoid fossa

Medial epicondyle

Trochlea

Radial notch of ulna

Coronoid process

Tuberosity of ulna

Radius

Ulna

(b) Posterior view

Medial epicondyle

Olecranon articulating with
olecranon fossa of humerus

Lateral epicondyle

Head of radius

Ulna

Radius

Figure 4 Bones of the right elbow and forearm

is the articulation between the capitulum and the head of the radius. The radiohumeral joint would be susceptible to dislocation if the thick annular ligament, which forms a ring around the proximal end of the radius, was not present to stabilize it. The third joint at the elbow, the proximal radioulnar joint, between the radial head and the ulnar notch, enables pronation – supination of the forearm and, therefore, repositions the hand about the long axis of the upper limb.

The elbow commonly suffers from overuse injury, particularly in racket or other hitting sports. The classic overuse injury of the elbow is lateral epicondylitis, also known as 'tennis elbow'. The injury is characterized by inflammation or degeneration of the tissues at the insertion of the wrist extensor tendons at the lateral epicondyle. Its occurrence is often linked to technical faults that result in excessive tension and stretch in the forearm muscles of the playing arm.

A common forehand fault that has been linked to tennis elbow is using wrist flexion and forearm supination to give the ball topspin, rather than moving the whole body and using shoulder power. A common backhand fault is using excessive elbow and wrist extension to give power to the shot. Using a double-handed backhand avoids this technique and emphasizes power from the trunk and shoulder. In addition to technique faults, equipment can also contribute to excessive loading of the extensor muscles of the forearm. Heavy rackets, particularly those with most of their weight in the head, increase the load on the muscles of the forearm in maintaining racket position. A racket with highly tensioned strings will results in more force being transmitted up the arm, rather than some of the contact force being dissipated in the racket itself. Finally, inappropriate grip size, either too large or too small, can contribute to the development of excess tension in the forearm.

Further reading

Perkins, R.H. and Davis, D. (2006) 'Musculoskeletal injuries in tennis', *Physical Medicine and Rehabilitation Clinics of North America*, 17: 609–31.

See also **elbow and forearm; elbow and forearm – bones; elbow and forearm – joints; elbow and forearm – ligaments; elbow and forearm – muscles.**

Elbow and forearm – ligaments

The elbow joint includes the ulnohumeral, radiohumeral and proximal radioulnar joints. This complex joint is held together by several extracapsular ligaments. On the sides of the joint are the medial and lateral collateral ligaments, which are also referred to as the ulnar and radial collateral ligaments. The medial collateral ligament runs from the medial humeral epicondyle to the coronoid process and olecranon of the ulna. The lateral collateral ligament runs from the lateral epicondyle of the humerus to the anular ligament. These two ligaments check movement of the ulnohumeral and radiohumeral joints in flexion and extension, as well as checking the small amount of abduction and adduction which occurs at the elbow.

The forearm is a unique structure because the two bones within it, the ulna and radius, are able to move from their normal side-by-side position to a crossed position. This movement is pronation – supination and is possible because of a special ligamentous structure around the head of the radius. The anular ligament is a ring of tissue which surrounds the head of the radius at the proximal end of the forearm. The proximal radioulnar joint is a pivot joint, meaning that the radius rotates about its long axis as the head rotates within the anular ligament. This movement, along with pivoting at the distal radioulnar joint, results in the radius crossing over the ulna as the forearm moves into pronation. There is an additional structure, the interosseous membrane, which provides further support to the bones of the forearm. The interosseous membrane runs the length of the shaft of the forearm bones, filling in the space between them.

See also **elbow and forearm; elbow and forearm – bones; elbow and forearm – joints; elbow and forearm – muscles.**

Elbow and forearm – muscles

The muscles of the elbow and forearm can be divided into five groups: the muscles of the arm that are involved with movements at the elbow joint, and four groups in the forearm. The forearm muscles are divided into anterior and posterior groups, and then subdivided further into superficial and deep groups. The muscles of the arm responsible for elbow flexion are: biceps brachii, the large muscle on the front of the arm; brachialis which is deep to biceps brachii; and brachioradialis, a smaller muscle that inserts into the base of the radial styloid process. The biceps also contributes to supination of the forearm and stabilizing the shoulder joint. Biceps is a weak shoulder flexor. The muscles arising from the medial epicondyle of the humerus are the superficial flexors of the forearm and can also contribute to elbow flexion. The extensors of the elbow are the triceps brachii on the back of the humerus and the small anconeus.

The superficial muscles on the anterior aspect of the forearm are the pronator teres, flexor carpi radialis, palmaris longus, flexor carpi ulnaris, and flexor digitorum superficialis, all of which originate from the medial humeral epicondyle at the elbow. These muscles act variously to pronate the forearm and to flex, abduct, and adduct the wrist (*see* **wrist and hand – muscles**). The deep anterior muscles of the forearm are the flexor digitorum profundus and flexor pollicis longus, which flex the fingers and thumb respectively. Additionally, pronator quadratus pronates the forearm.

The superficial muscles on the posterior aspect of the forearm originate on the lateral epicondyle. They are extensor carpi radialis longus, extensor carpi radialis brevis, extensor digitorum, extensor digiti minimi, and extensor carpi ulnaris. These muscles extend, abduct and adduct the wrist and extend the digits (*see* **wrist and hand – muscles**). The deep muscles of the posterior forearm are: supinator, which supinates the forearm; abductor pollicis longus, extensor pollicis brevis, extensor pollicis longus, which extend and abduct the thumb; and extensor indicis which extends the index finger.

The muscles of the elbow and forearm are at risk of both traumatic and overuse injury. Traumatic ruptures of the tendon of either biceps or triceps brachii are relatively uncommon, but may occur when large forces are exerted quickly on the tendon. An athlete will usually be able to recall a specific moment when the injury occurred. This injury is serious and requires surgical repair to give an athlete the best chance of regaining their pre-injury ability. Overuse injuries in this region are typically epicondylitis at the elbow, inflammation of the tendon attachments. Common examples are tennis elbow, or lateral epicondylitis (*see* **elbow and forearm – joints**), and golfer's elbow, or medial epicondylitis. These injuries are often due to errors in technique, making them particularly common in novice players.

See also **elbow and forearm; elbow and forearm – bones; elbow and forearm – joints; elbow and forearm – ligaments.**

Foot arches

The foot has three arches: the medial longitudinal arch, the shorter lateral longitudinal arch, and the transverse arch. These arches enable the foot to safely and effectively transmit large loads during contact with the ground. The bony structure of the foot and its soft tissues both contribute to the integrity of the foot arches. The plantar aponeurosis is the key soft tissue structure associated with them. This strong and wide band runs under the sole of the foot from the heel to the ball. Its connection to both the rear foot and forefoot helps to prevent the bony structure of the foot from collapsing when a downward vertical load is applied to it, as during weight bearing. Lack of appropriate soft tissue support causes the foot to be excessively flexible, reducing its effectiveness as a rigid lever when pushing off from the ground. This is commonly known as 'flat feet' or pes planus.

A common overuse injury associated with the arches of the feet is plantar fasciitis, caused by repetitive overload of the plantar aponeurosis. The symptoms are pain in the sole of the foot that is worse early in the morning and after excessive standing. This injury is often resolved by stretching of the plantar fascia and the Achilles tendon, lessening the tensile load on the fascia. Alternatively, it may be appropriate to support the foot using an orthotic device (*see* **Hot Topic 2**).

See also **ankle and foot; ankle and foot – bones; ankle and foot – joints; ankle and foot – ligaments; ankle and foot – muscles.**

Hot Topic 2: the use of foot orthotics in the prevention of injury

In-shoe foot orthotics are often prescribed to prevent overuse injuries in runners and other athletes, as well as in sedentary individuals who sustain an injury during their everyday activities. The purpose of a foot orthotic is to provide support for the foot and keep it in good alignment as weight is transferred onto the foot during walking and running. In many cases, orthotics are intended to provide support in the region of the medial longitudinal arch of a flat foot (*see* **foot arches**). Injuries thought to be related to an extremely pronated or flat foot position include plantar fasciitis and patellofemoral pain. Plantar fasciitis is a painful foot injury in which the insertion of the plantar fascia on the calcaneus (heel bone) becomes inflamed due to constant stretching of the plantar fascia. The plantar fascia is a key support structure for the medial longitudinal arch of the foot and is stretched when the foot pronates excessively and the arch collapses. The use of an orthotic can provide support for the arch and prevent this extreme position from being reached. This reduces the irritation of the insertion of the plantar fascia and may prevent the injury from recurring.

Patellofemoral pain is a knee injury where pain is felt behind the patella (kneecap). This injury is also thought to be related to excessive pronation of the foot. Excessive pronation of the foot may change the alignment of the entire lower limb, which can be thought of as a linked chain. Pronation of the foot is linked to internal rotation of the tibia, which may change the relationship between the femur and the patella via internal rotation of the femur. This knock-on effect would then alter the contact position and area between the patella and femur and lead to pain due to abnormal lateral tracking of the patella.

The research literature related to the effectiveness of orthotics in the treatment of pain and prevention of this type of injury is inconclusive. However, many people have great success in resolving their pain with orthotics. Part of the reason for the conflicting reports may be that there are so many types of orthotic available. Mass-produced off-the-shelf orthotics can be purchased cheaply, but may not suit the individual foot type or provide support in the right places. Orthotics can be custom made for the individual by a podiatrist or physiotherapist. In this case, the clinician makes a cast of the foot and then decides how much to reposition the foot, how much support to add, and whether to use flexible or rigid materials. Due to the custom nature of this type of orthotic, the cost is much higher.

Further reading

Collins, N., *et al.* (2007) 'Foot orthoses in lower limb overuse conditions: a systematic review and meta-analysis', *Foot and Ankle International*, 28: 396–412.

Gait analysis

Gait analysis is the study of walking or running. It is used in both clinical and sporting contexts and ranges from basic observational analysis to advanced three-dimensional motion analysis (*see* **Hot Topic 3**). Key components of the gait cycle are considered and the physiotherapist or sports scientist reports on these to the client, making comparisons with the normal gait cycle and focusing on those aspects that might be related to an increased risk of injury. The principles of gait analysis can be extended to general analysis of technique in different sports.

In the clinical domain, gait analysis is most commonly used in the treatment of children with cerebral palsy. Three-dimensional gait analysis is used as one of the decision-making tools in the surgical treatment of walking difficulties in this patient group. It is also used to provide an objective record of the effects of surgery, to aid the determination of the efficacy of different surgical procedures. These same tools are also used in sport by biomechanists who are interested in analyzing the movement of an athlete. Apart from its obvious application to runners and running injuries, gait analysis is also relevant to many other sports that have a large running component, such as team sports like soccer. The major difference between the two applications is that clinical analysis is concerned with basic walking ability whereas sports-related analysis usually focuses on running and the non-surgical correction of more minor biomechanical problems to reduce the risk of injury and enable the athlete to handle their desired training load successfully.

Gait analysis can be conducted at varying degrees of complexity, with more information being available as increasingly complex technology is introduced. The most basic form of gait analysis is observation. With practice, a trained eye can determine gross changes in an individual's gait pattern and locate the joint or segment of the body that is affected. This method is quick and requires no special equipment, so it is often used in a clinical environment where time and resources are limited. Observational gait analysis relies heavily on the skill and experience of the observer, and even then can only reveal major gait abnormalities.

The next stage of sophistication is qualitative video gait analysis, in which video cameras are used to record the gait of the individual in both the sagittal and frontal planes (*see* **planes and axes of movement**). The advantage of video analysis over simple observation is that a permanent record of gait is obtained, which can be returned to and reassessed at a future date, for example when comparing gait before and after a specific intervention designed to make changes and improve gait function. Video analysis also enables the gait cycle to be paused at any instant to study the position of the body in more detail. This ability to pause and play back the recorded movement at slow speeds is a huge advantage over observational analysis, as it often reveals movements that are either too subtle or occur too quickly to be registered by the naked eye. However, video analysis also has its limitations, the most significant of which is its two-dimensionality. Recording movement onto video necessarily projects a three-dimensional activity into two dimensions. Consequently, movements toward and away from the plane of view of the camera are difficult to detect and assess. This is partly overcome by the use of recordings in both the sagittal and frontal planes, but transverse plane rotations remain difficult to follow.

The most sophisticated type of gait analysis is a full three-dimensional kinematic and kinetic analysis of gait. Such an assessment requires sophisticated motion capture and force measuring equipment and is more time consuming, both in preparing participants for their gait to be recorded and during the data analysis and interpretation. Consequently, it is also more expensive, typically eight to ten times more costly than video analysis. However, as a result of its increased sophistication a three-dimensional gait analysis provides a lot of quantitative and objective information about the gait of an individual. All of this information can be interpreted by the skilled clinician or sports biomechanist and used as the basis for an assessment of the risk of injury owing to the gait pattern and any associated biomechanical abnormalities.

There is some evidence that intervening and altering an individual's gait through a series of gait retraining sessions can enable them to adjust their mechanics closer to the norm and, consequently, reduce their risk of injury through poor alignment of the lower body segments. This kind of gait retraining is currently the subject of research in sport and exercise biomechanics. In the future, gait-retraining clinics may be available for runners with recurrent injuries to attend and have their running mechanics adjusted as an accepted rehabilitation procedure.

The basic principles of gait analysis are to compare the movements of the individual to what is considered to be the norm for the general population. An acceptable range of normal motion is reported, to allow for the differing anatomical structure and anthropometry of individuals within the population, but the basics remain the same. The secret to a successful gait analysis is to identify the key movements, for example those that occur at initial foot contact, and determine the likely effect and possible causes of deviations from what is normal at that instant in the gait cycle. These principles can be extended to technique analysis in general and applied to many different sports activities, particularly those that require repeated stereotyped movements, for example, rowing and cycling.

Further reading

Perry, J. (1992) *Gait Analysis: Normal and Pathological Function*, Thorofare, NJ: SLACK Incorporated.

Whittle, M.W. (2001) *Gait Analysis: An Introduction*, Oxford: Butterworth Heinemann.

See also **qualitative and quantitative analysis of movement.**

Hot Topic 3: quantitative motion analysis in biomechanics

Quantitative motion analysis involves recording movement by tracking markers attached to the body. Biomechanists use quantitative motion analysis as a tool in human movement research. Kinematic and, when combined with use of force measurement, kinetic variables can be calculated from the output of the motion capture system. These systems enable the position of the markers, and hence the body segments to which they are attached, to be located accurately in three-dimensional space. Typically, the systems can do this to within 1 mm, so are very accurate. The systems work at a high frequency, taking between 60 and 240 samples every second, with the newest systems able to record up to 500 samples per second.

The space in which data are collected is known as the capture volume; it needs to be large enough to encompass the whole of the movement of interest, but not so long that large parts of the volume are unused. Six or more cameras will be used to cover a capture volume, although some multi-person motion captures in large volumes may use 24 or even 32 cameras. Generally, cameras are spaced equally around a volume to ensure maximum coverage and accuracy in marker position reconstruction.

Markers are placed on the participant at known anatomical landmarks that relate to the underlying skeletal structure. Typically 25 to 30 lightweight markers of between 10 mm and 25 mm in diameter are attached to the body at various locations. The most accurate way of tracking skeletal motion would be to use pins to attach markers directly to the bone, but this is obviously impractical for routine motion analysis, although it is used in some research studies. To reconstruct the position and orientation of a segment in three-dimensional space, at least three markers are required on every segment that is being tracked. Careful marker placement is very important, as it will directly affect the validity of the final results of the motion analysis. The results of an on-line motion analysis session carried out by a sports biomechanist are presented in an anatomically meaningful way (*see* **planes and axes of movement**) so that they can be understood by physiotherapists, coaches, and other personnel working with an athlete.

On-line motion analysis has the advantage of being able to provide accurate three-dimensional data quickly and easily with minimal processing time by the biomechanist. It is far less labor intensive than video analysis and the most advanced systems can produce graphical output of joint angles in real time, as the data are being collected. This real-time feedback has great potential in the development of rehabilitation strategies after injury and is actively being developed as an advanced clinical tool by biomechanics researchers. The main disadvantage of on-line motion capture is that it cannot be used in the field or in competition because it requires the application of markers to the performer's body and the cameras are unable to track markers outdoors. It is, however, a powerful tool for laboratory-based analysis.

Further reading

Milner, C.E. (2007) 'Motion analysis using online systems', in C. Payton and R. Bartlett (eds) *Biomechanical Analysis of Movement in Sport and Exercise: The British Association of Sport and Exercise Sciences Guide*, Oxon: Routledge.

Head and neck

The bones of the head and neck are those of the skull plus the seven cervical vertebrae. Most of the twenty-two bones of the skull are fused and form a strong protective case for the delicate tissues of the brain. The cervical vertebrae enable the neck to move in all three cardinal planes (*see* **planes and axes of movement**).

The skull is mainly at risk of traumatic injury owing to accidental contact with an opponent, sports equipment, or the ground. For example, if two players try to head the ball in a soccer match, they may accidentally hit each other and cause an injury such as a broken nose. Similarly, in squash, contact with the opponent's racket or the ball can lead to eye injuries. The neck and cervical spine are at risk of overuse injuries if extremes of head position are held for long periods. For example, cyclists may suffer from neck pain as a result of hyperextending the neck to lift the head sufficiently to see ahead. This overuse injury can be prevented by setting up the bicycle correctly, so that such an extreme position of the neck is not necessary for the cyclist to be able to see the road or track ahead.

See also **axial skeleton; head and neck – bones; head and neck – joints; head and neck – ligaments; head and neck – muscles.**

Head and neck – bones

The bones of the head and neck comprise the bones of the skull and the seven vertebrae of the cervical spine. The bones of the skull, which are fused in the adult, are the cranium – the large dome that houses and protects the brain – and the bones of the face (Figure 5). The skull is made up of eight cranial and fourteen facial bones. All of these, except the mandible (jawbone), are attached rigidly to each other by interlaced articulations called sutures. The bones of the skull are not fully fused at the sutures until old age and do not begin to close until about age 22 years, with the process being mostly complete by age 30.

This should be taken into consideration when younger athletes suffer a traumatic injury to the head, since the skull serves to protect the delicate tissues of the brain. Damage to the bones of the skull tends to be due to acute trauma from contact with another athlete, equipment, or the ground.

The cranial bones are the occipital bone at the back of the head, the two parietal bones forming the sides and top of the cranium, the frontal bone of the forehead, the two temporal bones at the sides below the parietal bones in the region of the ears, the sphenoid bone at the base of the skull extending laterally in front of the temporal bones, and the ethmoid bone that forms the walls of the superior part of the nasal cavity. The facial bones are the two nasal bones (the bridge of the nose), the two maxillae of the upper jaw, the palatine bone behind the maxillae (forming parts of the roof of the mouth), the floor of the nasal cavity, and the floor of the eye orbit, the two inferior nasal conchae (the lateral walls of the nasal cavity), the two vomers that are also part of the nasal cavity, the two lacrimal bones (part of the eye orbit), and the two zygomatic (cheek) bones.

Injuries to the head and neck tend to be traumatic and often occur as a result of unintentional contact between two players in team sports such as soccer. Typical injuries include nosebleeds, broken noses, concussion, and fracture of the facial bones, and may be severe enough to require hospitalization. In some sports, such as cycling, protective headgear can be worn to reduce the risk of severe head trauma in the case of unintentional contact with the ground.

Racket sports are the most common source of sports-related eye injuries. Squash is the biggest contributor, followed by badminton and then tennis. Such injuries are caused by the racket, shuttlecock, or ball. The best protection from these injuries is to wear eye guards that prevent objects from entering the eye from any angle.

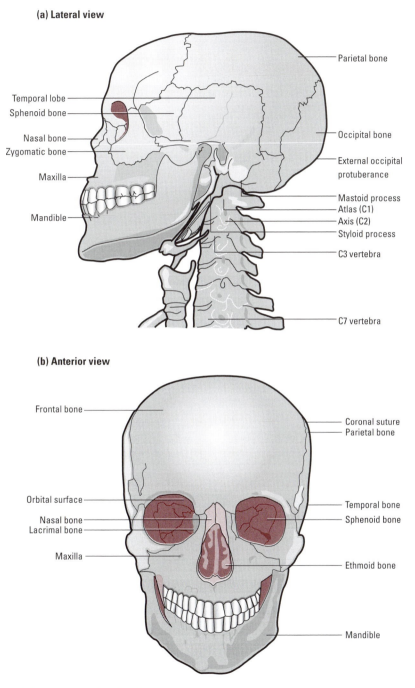

Figure 5 Bones of the head and neck

See also **bone; bone classification; head and neck; head and neck – joints; head and neck – ligaments; head and neck – muscles; vertebral structure.**

Head and neck – joints

Most bones of the head are rigidly attached to each other by interwoven articulations known as sutures. The only movable bone of the head is the mandible, or jawbone, which articulates with the temporal bones of the skull. The neck, containing the cervical spine, articulates with the cranium as well as adjacent vertebrae. The cervical spine carries the head and enables it to assume many different positions as a result of flexion – extension, axial rotation, and lateral flexion of the neck.

The two temporomandibular joints between the temporal bones of the skull and the jawbone are combined hinge and gliding joints. These joints enable the jaw to be opened and closed, protruded forward, and displaced laterally. In contact sports, such as boxing, the jaw is at risk of being broken or dislocated as a result of a direct blow to the face. This type of injury may also occur in contact team sports such as rugby.

The occipital bone of the skull rests on top of the first cervical vertebra, the atlas. The movements between these two bones are mainly flexion – extension; there is also a slight lateral motion of the head. Axial rotation of the atlas and, therefore, the skull, occurs at the joint between it and the axis – the second cervical vertebra. The joints between the individual vertebrae allow only a slight range of motion, but when the total for a region of the spine is added together, the range of motion is significant. The movements that can occur in the vertebral column are flexion – extension, lateral flexion, axial rotation, and circumduction. The largest range of motion is in flexion. All of these movements are greatest in the cervical spine, which is the most flexible part of the spinal column.

Overuse injuries to the joints can occur in the cervical region. Cyclists commonly suffer from such overuse injury. Neck pain can occur as a result of excessive hyperextension of the neck during cycling and typically affects the first three cervical vertebrae. The risk of overuse injury of the neck can be minimized by setting up the bicycle appropriately for the individual. Riding with the hands set too low in relation to the body, either by having the handlebars too low or spending too much time on the dropped part of the handlebar can contribute to this injury. Additionally, riding a bicycle that is too long and causes the rider to overreach will also put the rider in a disadvantageous position. Generally, raising the torso by attending to either of these set-up faults will resolve the neck pain.

General poor posture, in either everyday life or specific sports, can lead to neck pain. The cervical spine tends to be overloaded when other parts of the body are in poor alignment, because it is flexible and directly responsible for the position of the head.

See also head and neck; head and neck – bones; head and neck – ligaments; head and neck – muscles.

Head and neck – ligaments

The majority of bones in the head are fused to each other via sutures to provide a protective shell for the brain. Movement occurs at the temporomandibular joint, to allow opening and closing of the mouth. There are several ligaments associated with this joint. The joint capsule is thickened into a lateral ligament, sometimes referred to as the temporomandibular ligament. This ligament adds support to the lateral aspect of the joint and helps to prevent posterior dislocation. There are two additional ligaments extrinsic to the temporomandibular joint: the stylomandibular and sphenomandibular ligaments. These ligaments connect the mandible to points on the cranium. The stylomandibular ligament runs from the styloid process of the temporal cranial bone to the angle of the mandible distally. The sphenomandibular ligament runs from the spine of the sphenoid cranial bone to the lingula of the mandible, which is superior to the insertion of the stylomandibular ligament.

The neck is the most proximal part of the vertebral column, the cervical region. Therefore, it has several ligaments in common with the thoracic and lumbar regions of the spine. These common ligaments are the: anterior and posterior longitudinal ligaments, ligamentum flavum, interspinous and supraspinous ligaments (*see* **thoracic region – ligaments**). There is an additional ligament unique to the cervical region: the nuchal ligament. This ligament runs medially on the posterior aspect of the neck. Specifically, it runs from the external occipital protuberance and posterior border of the foramen magnum of the skull to the spinous processes of the cervical vertebrae. The spinous processes are short in the cervical region of the vertebral column, so the strong and thick nuchal ligament provides a substitute for muscular attachment in this region.

See also **head and neck; head and neck – bones; head and neck – joints; head and neck – muscles.**

Head and neck – muscles

Most muscles of the head and neck are involved in either facial expression or mastication (chewing) and are not directly involved in sports injuries, other than superficial bruising and contusions. The muscles of the neck, however, are heavily involved in sports activities because they are responsible for orienting the head via movements of the cervical spine.

The lateral muscles of the neck are the trapezius and the sternocleidomastoid. Similarly to the muscles on either side of the lumbar spine (*see* **lumbar spine and pelvis – muscles**), the action of the sternocleidomastoid muscles depends on whether one or both of them are active. Contraction of the muscle on one side of the head bends the neck laterally to the same side or rotates the head towards the opposite side. The action of both muscles together flexes the neck forwards.

The trapezius is a large muscle that acts at the shoulder as well as the neck (*see* **shoulder complex – muscles**). Its role at the neck is to draw the neck towards the side that is contracting, while turning the face away from that side; trapezius extends the neck if both sides contract simultaneously.

Deep muscles attached directly to the vertebral column are also responsible for movements of the neck. Anteriorly on the neck, longus colli, longus capitis, and anterior rectus capitis contribute to forward flexion, and lateral rectus capitis flexes the neck laterally towards the side that is contracting. Posteriorly, the deep muscles of the back are responsible for extension of the vertebral column. At the cervical level, the deep muscles responsible for neck extension and rotation are splenius cervicis, iliocostalis cervicis, longissimus capitis, spinalis capitis, and semispinalis capitis.

The neck can be subject to both overuse and traumatic injury. Sports that require the neck to be held in the same extreme position for extended periods are prone to overuse injury as a result of the excess loading placed on the muscles involved. Examples of such injuries can be found in cycling, where the neck may be hyperextended to enable the eyes to look directly forwards (*see* **head and neck – joints**).

Strengthening the neck may protect it from traumatic injury caused by movements at the extremes of its range of motion. This type of injury is a particular risk in contact sports, such as wrestling and rugby, in which the neck may be in close contact with either an opponent or the ground. Neck strength can be increased by various means. For example, harnesses with weights attached can be worn hanging from the head to provide extra resistance for flexion and extension movements. These isolation exercises work specifically on neck strength but may not replicate very closely what happens during the sports activity. Various bridging exercises, in which athletes lie supine and then raise themselves up on to the top of the head and the soles of the feet while arching the back – followed by lowering the body under control – also strengthen the neck. The advantage of these exercises is that they also recruit the smaller stabilizing muscles of the head and neck region and improve both strength and awareness of body position that are vital to minimizing the risk of injury in sports.

See also **head and neck; head and neck bones; head and neck – joints; head and neck – ligaments.**

Hip

The hip joint is formed between the acetabulum of the hip bone in the pelvis, and the proximal end of the femur. The hip is the most mobile joint of the lower extremity and is able to rotate about all three axes (*see* **planes and axes of movement**) owing to its configuration as a ball and socket joint (*see* **joints**). The hip is a stable joint with many strong ligamentous attachments that contribute to its stability, in addition to its bony structure. As a result, it is dislocated much less frequently than its upper extremity equivalent, the glenohumeral (shoulder) joint (*see* **shoulder complex – joints**).

However, as a result of its structure and large ranges of motion in all three cardinal planes, the hip is implicated in overuse injuries of the lower extremities. For example, it is relatively common for runners, particularly females, to run with the hip joint excessively internally rotated. Although the hip joint is easily able to accommodate this, rotation at the joint changes the alignment of the whole lower extremity, the distal joints of which are less able to adapt to the change. This places bony and soft tissue structures under increased loads as they try to accommodate the alignment at the hip alongside the constraints of foot contact with the ground during the gait cycle. Over the many repetitions of many miles of running during training and competition, this malalignment increases wear and tear on the tissues of the lower extremity and may lead to overuse injury. Despite the movement changes being at the hip, injury often occurs more distally in the lower extremity, at the knee.

See also **hip; hip – bones; hip – joint; hip – ligaments; hip – muscles.**

Hip – bones

The hip is the most proximal joint of the lower extremity and has the greatest multiaxial range of motion of all the lower extremity joints. It is formed between the hip bone, which is part of the pelvis and consists of the ilium, ischium and pubis, and the femur, the long bone between the hip and the knee (Figure 6). The hip is a ball and socket joint (*see* **joints**) and, as such, makes the thigh and lower limb very mobile with respect to the pelvis. Because of its bony configuration, the joint is stabilized by both the cup-like acetabulum of the hip bone and the strong ligamentous attachments between it and the femur.

The femur has a long and cylindrical diaphysis. Proximally, it has a short neck inclined to the long axis of the bone and an approximately spherical head that sits in the acetabulum of the pelvis. Distally, the femur thickens into the femoral condyles that make up the proximal part of the knee joint. Differences in the bony anatomy of the femur can affect lower extremity movements and, like other lower limb structural abnormalities, are thought to be related to the incidence of overuse injuries of the lower extremity.

The major structural abnormalities of the femur are femoral anteversion and large Q angle. The Q angle expresses the geometric relationship between the pelvis, femur, patella, and tibia in the frontal plane. It is measured as the acute angle between a line drawn from the anterior superior iliac spine of the pelvis to the centre of the patella and a line drawn from the centre of the patella to the tibial tuberosity. It provides an indication of the medial angulation of the femur between the hip joint and the knee joint, which accommodates the difference between the width of the pelvis and the base of support at the feet. This angle is typically higher in women as a result of their wider pelvis relative to femur length. The Q angle is one of the structural measures that have been investigated by sports biomechanists in an attempt to determine the cause of lower extremity overuse injuries, such as those that occur during running.

Femoral anteversion is medial torsion of the femur, the internal rotation of the distal end of the femur relative to the proximal end (*see* **planes and axes of movement**). This changes the alignment of the bones at the knee and can lead to knee overuse injuries caused by malalignment of the femur relative to the patella and tibia, such as

(a) Anterior view

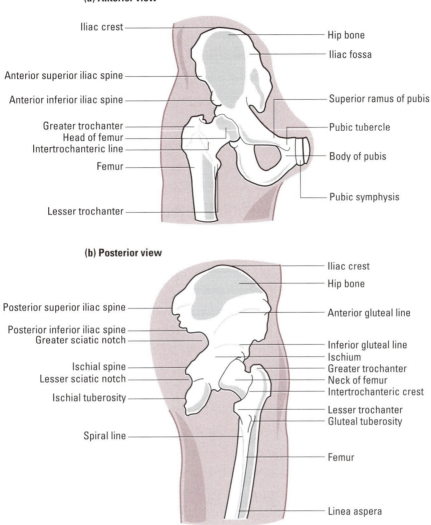

Iliac crest

Hip bone

Iliac fossa

Anterior superior iliac spine

Anterior inferior iliac spine

Superior ramus of pubis

Greater trochanter
Head of femur
Intertrochanteric line

Pubic tubercle

Femur

Body of pubis

Pubic symphysis

Lesser trochanter

(b) Posterior view

Iliac crest

Hip bone

Posterior superior iliac spine

Anterior gluteal line

Posterior inferior iliac spine
Greater sciatic notch

Inferior gluteal line
Ischium
Greater trochanter
Neck of femur
Intertrochanteric crest

Ischial spine
Lesser sciatic notch

Ischial tuberosity

Lesser trochanter
Gluteal tuberosity

Spiral line

Femur

Linea aspera

Figure 6 Bones of the right hip

chondromalacia patella. Observing the static standing posture of an individual can identify femoral anteversion; the patella, or kneecap, is turned inwards instead of pointing straight ahead, and the toes are often turned in too. It is possible to correct the anteversion of the femur surgically, although this is only considered if the anteversion is severe enough to interfere with daily activities.

Typical overuse injuries that occur in runners and which might be related to femoral anteversion or the Q angle include chondromalacia patella, patellofemoral pain, iliotibial band friction syndrome, and tibial and femoral stress fractures (*see* **Hot Topic 1**).

See also **bone; bone classification; hip; hip – joint; hip – ligaments; hip – muscles; lumbar spine and pelvis – muscles.**

Hip – joint

The hip joint is formed between the femur and the hip bone of the pelvis. The hip bone consists of the ilium, ischium, and pubis, which are fused. Both hip bones, along with the sacrum and coccyx of the spine, form the pelvis. Therefore, the hip joint is the link between the pelvis in the torso and the thigh in the lower extremity. The femur is held firmly in place by strong ligaments and the joint capsule. The hip is a ball and socket joint (*see* **joints**), with the head of the femur fitting into the acetabulum of the hip bone, and is the most mobile joint of the lower extremity. Movements at the hip are sagittal plane flexion – extension, frontal plane abduction – adduction, and transverse plane internal – external rotation (*see* **planes and axes of movement**).

Because of its high mobility, malalignment of the hip joint can occur during running. This may lead to overuse injuries of the lower extremity because poor alignment at the hip will result in adaptations further down the kinetic chain between the hip and the ground. Incorrect alignment of the lower extremity changes the distribution of load in the bony and soft tissue structures; this is particularly significant as loads of up to three times body weight are transmitted up the lower extremity with each foot strike during running. When we consider that there are around 500 foot strikes with each limb during every kilometre run, it is easy to appreciate how these small changes can become significant. Common alignment problems at the hip include excessive adduction and excessive internal rotation. Excessive hip adduction is usually due to the pelvis dropping on the contralateral (opposite) side during the stance phase of gait. This may be due to weakness in the antagonist hip abductor muscles, but may also be due to a lack of stability in the lower torso, commonly known as **core stability.**

See also **hip; hip – bones; hip – ligaments; hip – muscles; joint classification; lumbar spine and pelvis – muscles.**

Hip – ligaments

The hip is a very stable joint, with stability provided by the ball and socket configuration of the femur and pelvic bones and several thick and strong ligaments. There are three ligaments external to the hip joint: the iliofemoral, ischiofemoral, and pubofemoral ligaments. They are named according to the parts of the hip bone that they are attached to, plus their attachment to the femur. There are two more ligaments at the hip inside the ball and socket of the joint: the ligament of the head of the femur and the transverse acetabular ligament. The ligament of the femoral head directly attaches the head of the femur to the acetabulum of the hip bone. There is a small pit in the smooth head of the femur, the fovea, where the ligament attaches. Similarly, the other end of the ligament attaches to the center of the acetabular fossa, where it is surrounded by the smooth lunate surface of the acetabulum. This internal hip joint ligament prevents the head of the femur from rotating too far in any direction within the acetabulum. The transverse acetabular ligament helps to make the socket of the hip joint deeper, along with the acetabular labrum, a rim of fibrocartilage around the edge of the acetabulum. The ligament crosses the acetabular notch, part of the rim not extended by the labrum, making a complete ring of soft tissue. As a result of this extension of the acetabulum, more than half of the femoral head fits within the socket of the hip joint.

As a synovial joint (*see* **joint classification**), the hip joint is surrounded by a fibrous capsule. Thickenings of this capsule form the three external ligaments of the hip. These ligaments spiral from the pelvis to the femur, providing strong support for the joint. The most anterior ligament is the iliofemoral ligament, also known as the Y-ligament because it has a characteristic inverted Y-shape. This ligament arises from the anterior inferior iliac spine and acetabular rim of the pelvis, winding anteriorly and distally to attach at two points on the intertrochanteric line on the proximal anterior femur. The major role of this ligament is to prevent hyperextension of the hip joint. The pubofemoral ligament has an anteroinferior position. It attaches to the obturator crest, laterally on the pubic bone, and runs laterally and distally to blend with the iliofemoral ligament at its femoral attachment. This ligament prevents excessive abduction of the hip joint. The third capsular ligament lies posterior to the hip joint. The ischiofemoral ligament arises from the ischial part of the rim of the acetabulum, spiraling proximally and laterally to attach to the superior surface of the neck of the femur, just medial to the greater trochanter. This ligament is the weakest of the three. All of the ligaments become tighter during hip extension, preventing hyperextension and pushing the head of the femur into the acetabulum and maximizing the stability of the joint.

Due to the high degree of stability at the hip joint provided by these strong ligaments which surround the joint, as well as the bony structure of the femur and hip bone, the hip joint is rarely dislocated. This is in contrast to the equivalent upper extremity joint, the glenohumeral joint at the shoulder (*see* **shoulder complex – joints**), which is the most commonly dislocated joint in the body. Both are ball and socket joints, but the glenohumeral joint has a much shallower socket. Since the hip must support and transfer the weight of the entire upper body to the lower extremities during standing and locomotion, this stability is an important feature.

See also **hip; hip – bones; hip – joint; hip – muscles; lumbar spine and pelvis – muscles.**

Hip – muscles

The muscles of the thigh can be divided broadly into the anterior femoral muscles on the front of the thigh, and the medial femoral and posterior femoral muscles on the medial side and back of the thigh respectively. These muscles have actions at both the knee (*see* **knee – muscles**) and the hip. This section will focus on the role of the muscles of the thigh in hip rotations. It should be noted that the gluteal muscles (*see* **lumbar spine and pelvis – muscles**) also contribute to movements at the hip joint.

The muscles on the front of the thigh are the quadriceps femoris group and the sartorius. The quadriceps femoris group consists of rectus femoris, vastus lateralis, vastus medialis, and vastus intermedius. As a whole, the group extends the knee; rectus femoris also flexes the hip. The major action of sartorius is hip flexion and external rotation. It also contributes to knee flexion and internal rotation.

As a group, the medial thigh muscles, gracilis, pectineus, and adductors longus, brevis, and magnus act at the hip. Gracilis adducts the thigh (*see* **planes and axes of movement**), and also has a role in knee flexion and internal rotation. Pectineus and the adductors act to flex and adduct the thigh and rotate it internally, although the lower portion of adductor magnus acts to extend the hip and externally rotate it.

The posterior femoral muscles, also known as the hamstrings, also act at both the knee and the hip. Biceps femoris extends the hip and externally rotates it. This muscle also flexes and externally rotates the knee. Semitendinosus also extends the hip and flexes the knee. Additionally, it contributes to internal rotation at the knee. Semimembranosus extends the hip and flexes and internally rotates the knee.

Given their major contribution to controlling rotations at both the hip and the knee joint, the muscles of the thigh have an important stabilization role during dynamic movements involving the lower extremity. As such, it is important that they are sufficiently strong to fulfill this role and protect and stabilize the joints against the large forces to which they are subjected in sports activities. Examples of compound exercises that engage the muscles of the thigh in their roles at both the hip and the knee are squats, dead lifts, and leg presses.

See also **hip; hip – bones; hip – joint; hip – ligaments; knee; knee – joint.**

Joint classification

Joints can be classified according to their structure or function. Classifying joints by structure, there are three major categories: fibrous, cartilaginous, and synovial. There are three subtypes of fibrous joint: sutures, syndesmoses, and gomphoses, and two subtypes of cartilaginous joint: synchondroses and symphyses. Fibrous joints are those in which the articulating bones are connected by fibrous connective tissue. There is no joint space or cavity and the joint is either immovable or only slightly movable. The three subtypes of fibrous joints differ in the types of articulation that they make. Sutures are found where the bones of the skull come together. They are the wavy interlocking edges of the skull bones (*see* **head and neck – bones**). The skull is made up of several interlocking bones, which allows for skull growth during childhood when the bones are still separate. The bones are tightly bound together by fibrous connective tissue and minimal movement occurs between them. The primary role of the bones of the skull is to protect the brain. The individual bones eventually fuse together during middle age. A gomphosis is another specialized type of fibrous joint. It is a peg-in-socket type of articulation, with the roots of the teeth being the pegs and the jaw bones containing the sockets. The periodontal ligament holds the tooth in the jaw bone and movement is minimal. The third type of fibrous joint is a syndesmosis, and is simply two bones connected by ligaments. The amount of movement possible at this type of joint depends on the length of the ligament. For example, the inferior anterior tibiofibular ligament, between the two leg bones just above the ankle, is short and only a small amount of 'give' is possible between the bones (*see* **ankle and foot – ligaments**). In contrast, the interosseous membrane in the forearm has longer fibers which allow free movement between the radius and ulna as the forearm pronates and supinates (*see* **elbow and forearm – joints**).

Cartilaginous joints are those in which the articulating bones are connected by cartilage. They do not have a joint cavity. The amount of movement possible at cartilaginous joints varies from immovable to highly movable, with synchondroses being immovable and symphyses being slightly or highly movable. A synchondrosis is a joint where the bones are firmly connected by hyaline cartilage (*see* **articulating surfaces**). Examples include the epiphyseal (growth) plates in the long bones of the extremities and sternocostal synchondroses between the sternum (breastbone) and the anterior end of the ribs in the thoracic cage (*see* **thoracic region – joints**). The second type of cartilaginous joint is a symphysis, in which the bones are connected by fibrocartilage. In these joints, hyaline cartilage is present on the articulating parts of the bone. These joints are somewhat movable and include the intervertebral joints. The fibrocartilaginous intervertebral disc connects the vertebral bodies and acts as a shock absorber within the vertebral column (*see* **thoracic region – joints**). Another example is the pubic symphysis on the anterior aspect of the pelvis (*see* **lumbar spine and pelvis – bones**). This joint becomes quite flexible prior to childbirth to enable the infant to pass more easily through the birth canal.

The third type of joint is a synovial joint. In this joint, articular cartilage is present on the bony surfaces, the bones are connected by ligaments and the joint is surrounded by a joint capsule. This type of joint is the most movable and is the most common type of joint, especially in the limbs. Examples of synovial joints include the knee, hip, and elbow joints.

Joints can also be categorized according to their function. There is some overlap here with the divisions according to structure. Synarthrodial joints are immovable and include sutures and gomphoses. Amphiarthrodial joints are slightly movable and include syndesmoses and synchondroses. Diarthrodial joints are freely movable and equate to synovial joints.

See also **ankle and foot – joints; articulating surfaces; elbow and forearm – joints; head and neck – joints; hip – joint; joints; knee – joints; lumbar spine and pelvis – joints; shoulder complex – joints; thoracic region – joints; wrist and hand – joints.**

Joints

Joints are also known as articulations. A joint is the junction between two or more bones. Typically joints are found at the ends of long bones. In short and irregular bones, joints are found wherever a bone touches another bone. The primary function of joints is to permit movement between the adjacent bones. However, not all joints are movable. The amount of movement possible at a joint varies from it being freely movable to only a small amount of movement permitted to no movement whatsoever between adjacent bones (*see* **joint classification**).

The freely movable synovial (diarthrodial) joints can be classified according to their structure. At the simplest level, synovial joints fit into one of two groups: simple or compound. A simple joint has only two **articulating surfaces**, one on each of the two bones that are touching. Compound joints have more than two articulating surfaces. For example at the knee (tibiofemoral joint) there are four articulating surfaces on two bones. At the elbow, three bones articulate with each other. Synovial joints can also be classified according to the shapes of the articulating surfaces. There are six different types of synovial joint according to their shape: ball and socket, gliding, ellipsoidal, hinge, saddle, and pivot joints.

A ball and socket (enarthrodial) joint consists of a bone with a ball-shaped head that sits in a cup-shaped cavity. This type of joint is highly mobile and allows movement about all three axes (*see* **planes and axes of movement**). Examples are the hip and shoulder joints. The hip has a deep socket and good bony stability, whereas the shoulder (glenohumeral) joint has a large ball and shallow socket. This gives it less bony stability, but allows a greater range of motion. Ellipsoidal (condyloidal) joints consist of a bone with an egg-shaped articular surface and a bone with an oval cavity. This type of joint is biaxial, allowing movement about two of the three axes. No rotation is possible about the long axis of the bone in this case. Examples include the wrist complex and the metacarpophalangeal joints (knuckles). Another type of biaxial joint is a saddle (sellar) joint. In this case, each joint has perpendicular concave and convex areas, like a horse saddle. Again, there is no rotation about the long axis in this joint. This type of joint is less common than the ellipsoidal joint; the first carpometacarpal joint is an example. A hinge joint is found between a bone with a cylindrical articular surface and a bone with a trough-shaped cavity. This joint is uniaxial, allowing movement about only one axis. Movement at this joint is planar (i.e. occurs in only one plane – that perpendicular to the axis of rotation). Examples include the ankle (talocrural), elbow (ulnohumeral), and finger (interphalangeal) joints. A pivot (trochoidal) joint is a special type of uniaxial joint. In this case, a bone with a rounded end is encircled by a ring formed from the second bone and its ligament: rotation is possible about the long axis of the encircled bone only. Pivot joints in the body are the proximal radioulnar and atlantoaxial joints. The least mobile type of synovial joint is a gliding (arthrodial) joint. This joint has flat articular surfaces and only allows short gliding or sliding movements between them. Examples include intervertebral, intertarsal, and intercarpal joints.

See also **ankle and foot – joints; articulating surfaces; elbow and forearm – joints; head and neck – joints; hip – joint; joint classification; knee – joints; lumbar spine and pelvis – joints; thoracic region – joints; wrist and hand – joints.**

Knee

The knee joint consists of the tibiofemoral joint, which is formed between the distal end of the femur and the proximal end of the tibia, and the patellofemoral joint, between the distal end of the femur and the patella, or kneecap. The major movement at the knee is sagittal plane flexion – extension (*see* **planes and axes of movement**), with lesser movements in the two secondary planes: abduction – adduction in the frontal plane and internal – external rotation in the transverse plane.

The knee is at risk of both traumatic and overuse injury owing to its structure. The bony surfaces do not provide much stability at the joint. Therefore, the knee relies on soft tissue structures – the cruciate ligaments, collateral ligaments, and menisci – to maintain the joint's integrity. Ligamentous injuries, such as anterior cruciate ligament rupture, at the knee are common and often result in residual instability, even after recovery and rehabilitation (*see* **Hot Topic 4**). In individuals who fail to recover fully from a soft tissue injury to the knee, a lack of proprioception often leads to feelings of insecurity about landing, hopping, or jumping with the leg injured previously. The knee may also suffer from unpredictable episodes of 'giving way', which add to feelings of insecurity about relying on that knee. However, this loose-packed arrangement of the joint enables some movement to occur about all three cardinal axes of rotation (*see* **planes and axes of movement**).

See also **knee – bones; knee – joints; knee – ligaments; knee – muscles.**

Knee – bones

The knee joint has a large sagittal plane range of motion (flexion – extension; *see* **planes and axes of movement**). The joint is formed between the two major long bones of the lower limb: the tibia, lying between the knee and the ankle, and the femur, lying between the knee and the hip. Although the fibula contributes to the ankle joint, it is not part of the knee joint. However, there is a third bone present at the knee, the patella (kneecap), which forms the patellofemoral joint by running along the intertrochanteric groove in the femur (Figure 7). Stabilization of the joint is predominantly by soft tissue structures: the anterior and posterior cruciate ligaments, the medial and lateral collateral ligaments, and the medial and lateral menisci. The distal end of the femur – the femoral condyles – rests on the flattened tibial plateau.

The primary knee joint axis runs in a mediolateral direction, although its absolute position varies with knee flexion. There are also lesser amounts of rotation in the two secondary planes, with abduction and adduction occurring around the anteroposterior axis and internal and external rotation occurring around the longitudinal axis of the tibia. Historically, these secondary planes of motion have been considered insignificant in the investigation of the cause of overuse injury at the knee. However, as sports biomechanists have access to more advanced equipment for on-line motion analysis, more research is focusing on these subtle joint movements. It is hypothesized that slight malalignments in the bones of the lower limb may change the amount and pattern of motion around the secondary axes of rotation at the knee and that these small changes, when repeated over the thousands of repetitions that occur during walking, running, or other activities may contribute to the development of overuse injuries at the joint.

Malalignment of the bones at the knee can lead to osteoarthritic deterioration of the condyles of the joint, with varus (adduction) alignment leading to deterioration of the medial compartment and valgus (abduction) alignment leading to deterioration of the lateral compartment. Biomechanics researchers are interested in conservative measures to improve the functional ability of individuals with knee osteoarthritis, such as in-shoe orthotics to improve the alignment of the bones at the knee joint and reduce the pressure on the arthritic side (*see* **Hot Topic 2**). These measures can improve the quality of life and

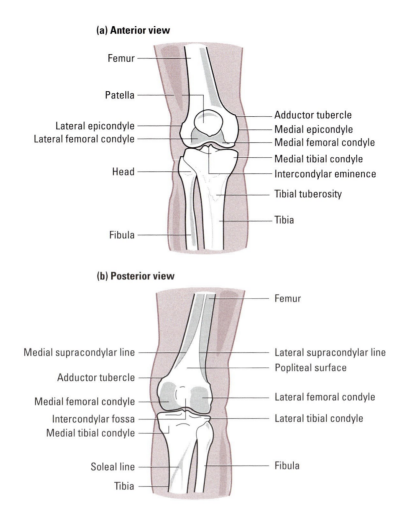

(a) Anterior view

Femur

Patella

Lateral epicondyle
Lateral femoral condyle

Head

Fibula

Adductor tubercle
Medial epicondyle
Medial femoral condyle
Medial tibial condyle
Intercondylar eminence

Tibial tuberosity

Tibia

(b) Posterior view

Femur

Medial supracondylar line

Lateral supracondylar line
Popliteal surface

Adductor tubercle

Medial femoral condyle

Lateral femoral condyle

Intercondylar fossa
Medial tibial condyle

Lateral tibial condyle

Soleal line

Fibula

Tibia

Figure 7 Bones of the right knee

the ability to remain physically active of an osteoarthritic individual, delaying or possibly removing the need for surgery. If knee osteoarthritis progresses beyond the limit at which these conservative measures can provide relief, total knee joint replacement is the surgical option. This involves replacing the distal end of the femur and the proximal end of the tibia with metal and polyethylene components. The prosthesis typically lasts for fifteen years and individuals can return to most sports activities, even skiing, after recovery from surgery.

See also **bone; bone classification; knee; knee – joints; knee – ligaments; knee – muscles.**

Knee – joints

The knee consists of the tibiofemoral joint between the long bones of the lower extremity, where the femoral condyles articulate with the tibial plateau. The patellofemoral joint lies between the intertrochanteric groove of the femur and the patella (kneecap). The tibiofemoral joint accommodates the movements that occur at the knee. The primary movement is flexion – extension in the sagittal plane (*see* **planes and axes of movement**). Typically, the knee has a range of motion of about 140° of flexion-extension, from about 5° of hyperextension to 135° of flexion. Secondary movements at the knee are abduction – adduction and internal – external rotation.

The significance of the secondary planes of motion at the knee joint is currently of interest to biomechanics researchers who are trying to determine the causes of overuse injuries to the knee, such as patellofemoral pain and iliotibial band syndrome. Although the movements in the secondary planes are smaller than the flexion – extension motion, when minor deviations in these movements are repeated over and over, as in walking or running, the effects may accumulate and contribute to overuse injury. Other factors thought to be related to overuse injuries at the knee are malalignment at the hip joint or in the foot.

The knee joint is susceptible to traumatic ligament tears because it relies on soft tissue and not bony structures for its stability. The most common acute injury at the knee joint is a tear of the anterior cruciate ligament (ACL: *see* **Hot Topic 4**).

It should be noted that the terms flexion and extension at the knee refer to rotation in the opposite direction about the mediolateral axis of the joint than at other joints. Flexion is generally the sagittal plane rotation that brings the distal segment towards the proximal segment anteriorly about the mediolateral axis in the **anatomical position**. However, flexion of the knee, brought about mainly by the hamstrings on the back of the thigh, is movement of the leg towards the hamstrings posteriorly. Contrast this with flexion of the hip by rectus femoris on the front of the thigh: movement of the thigh towards the front of the thorax.

See also **bone; bone classification; knee; knee – bones; knee – joints; knee – ligaments; knee – muscles.**

Knee – ligaments

The knee relies heavily on its ligaments for stability, since the bones themselves are somewhat flat in the area of contact. There are four major ligaments at the tibiofemoral joint, plus the menisci, additional soft tissue structures that also provide stability at the knee. The patellofemoral joint has one ligament associated with it: the patellar ligament.

The four ligaments associated with the tibiofemoral joint are in two pairs. Inside the joint are the anterior and posterior cruciate ligaments (ACL, PCL), and outside the joint are the medial and lateral collateral ligaments (MCL, LCL). Each ligament checks extremes of different rotations at the knee, according to its orientation and attachments. The ACL is the most commonly injured knee ligament in athletes, and is typically injured in a non-contact situation (*see* **Hot Topic 4**). The two cruciate ligaments are so named because they run on opposite diagonals in the middle of the knee joint, crossing over each other and making an X-shape. The ACL runs in a posterolateral direction from the anterior portion of the intercondylar area of the tibia to the medial side of the lateral femoral condyle. The PCL runs anteromedially from the posterior part of the tibial intercondylar area to the lateral side of the medial condyle of the femur. The primary roles of the ACL and PCL are to prevent anterior and posterior sliding of the tibia respectively. Since the tibial plateau is relatively flat, this is important in maintaining the integrity of the joint when muscle action tends to translate the tibia on the femur. The cruciate ligaments also check axial rotation of the tibia, with the ACL checking internal rotation and the PCL external rotation.

The MCL and LCL ligaments lie outside the joint capsule on the medial and lateral aspects of the knee. The MCL runs from the medial epicondyle of the femur to the medial condyle of the tibia and the LCL runs from the lateral epicondyle of the femur to the head of the fibula. Together these two ligaments check hyperextension of the knee. Individually, the MCL and LCL prevent excessive abduction and adduction of the knee respectively. Injury to these ligaments typically occurs in sports activities as a result of a contact injury. For example, the LCL could be injured during a heavy tackle from the side in rugby when the legs of the player being tackled are obstructed and prevented from moving with the tackle by a teammate lying on the ground. As the tackler moves the upper body of the player sideways, the knee is adducted. If the large force being applied during the tackle is greater than the tensile strength of the LCL, the ligament will rupture. At the moment the ligament ruptures, a loud pop is often heard as the ligament snaps. The result is an immediate loss of stability at the knee, allowing it to move into an extreme adducted position. The damaged ligament is typically surgically repaired or reconstructed in athletes to enable them to regain stability and return to play after a lengthy rehabilitation period.

In addition to these ligaments, the medial and lateral tibial condyles each have a meniscus. This is a C-shaped ring of fibrocartilage around the edge of each condyle which helps to deepen the tibial plateau and provide additional support and stability at the joint. The menisci increase the contact area between the femur and tibia, helping to distribute the loads transmitted through the knee more evenly.

Finally, the patellofemoral joint also has a ligament. This joint is different than the tibiofemoral joint because the patella is a sesamoid bone: a bone that lies within a tendon. The patella lies within the tendon of the powerful quadriceps muscle. This tendon crosses the knee joint to attach to the tibia; the patella improves the mechanical advantage of the quadriceps by moving the tendon further away from the center of the knee joint. The portion of tendon between the quadriceps muscle and the patella is called the quadriceps tendon and the portion below the patella that inserts onto the tibial tuberosity is the patellar tendon.

See also **knee; knee – bones; knee – joints; knee – muscles.**

Knee – muscles

The muscles of the knee are responsible for flexion and extension of the joint and for dynamic stabilization of the joint during activity. Therefore, these muscles work eccentrically and isometrically as well as concentrically (*see* **muscle contraction – types**). The muscle group on the front of the thigh, the quadriceps femoris, is responsible for extension of the knee joint; the muscle group on the back of the thigh, the hamstrings, is responsible for knee flexion. Other muscles of the lower limb play minor roles in the control of the knee joint. The role of the knee joint during gait provides a good example of the multifunctional roles of the muscles of the knee, with the muscles undergoing concentric and eccentric contraction during various phases of the gait cycle.

The quadriceps femoris muscle group – the rectus femoris, vastus lateralis, vastus medialis, and vastus intermedius – performs knee extension. The hamstrings – the long and short head of the biceps femoris, plus semitendinosus and semimembranosus – carry out flexion. Popliteus is a small muscle that flexes and internally rotates the knee. The gastrocnemius of the leg also has a flexing action on the knee, but its major role at the knee is preventing hyperextension of the knee joint. Gastrocnemius also plantarflexes the ankle (*see* **ankle and foot – muscles**).

During gait, these muscle groups act both concentrically and eccentrically. During the stance phase of gait the knee is flexed. However, there is a tendency for the knee to continue to flex and, ultimately, collapse under the weight of the body. To prevent this, the quadriceps muscle group acts eccentrically to restrict the knee flexion that occurs and ensure that the stance leg is stable while the whole of the body's weight is on it during single limb stance. Similarly, at the end of the swing phase of gait, when the knee is extending to place the foot in front of the body at heel strike, the hamstrings are acting eccentrically to slow the speed at which the knee is extending and prevent hyperextension of the joint from occurring. The hamstrings act concentrically at the end of the stance phase and beginning of the swing phase of gait to flex the knee in preparation for the swing limb moving forward past the stance limb.

The muscles of the knee provide support for the joint during dynamic activity. Since the knee joint is stabilized by soft tissue structures rather than its bony architecture, it is vital that these muscles have sufficient strength to support the joint during sporting activities. To isolate these specific muscle groups, single joint exercises should be used. For example, the seated knee extension exercise isolates the quadriceps muscle group, whereas the standing or lying hamstring curl isolates the hamstrings. However, the muscle groups rarely work in isolation in a sports movement, so compound or multijoint exercises reflect the functional role of the muscles more appropriately. Examples of compound exercises that work the muscles of the knee include squats of all types, dead lifts, leg presses, and power cleans.

Further reading

Perry, J. (1992) *Gait Analysis: Normal and Pathological Function*, Thorofare, NJ: SLACK Incorporated.

Whittle, M.W. (2001) *Gait Analysis: An Introduction*, Oxford: Butterworth Heinemann.

See also **gait analysis; knee; knee – bones; knee – joints; knee – ligaments.**

Hot Topic 4: anterior cruciate ligament injury in athletes

The anterior cruciate ligament (ACL) is the most commonly injured knee ligament in athletes. The knee is vulnerable to ligament injury because the bone structure does not provide much stability. The rounded condyles of the femur sit on the relatively flat tibial plateau (*see* **knee – bones**). Additional support is provided at the joint by the menisci and the cruciate and collateral ligaments (*see* **knee – ligaments**). The ACL is the primary restraint against anterior tibial displacement and internal rotation of the tibia at the knee. Non-contact ACL injuries occur when a high force at the joint in the direction of either internal rotation or anterior tibial translation exceeds the tensile strength of the ligament. Typically this occurs during landing from a jump or cutting in sports such as basketball, soccer, and volleyball. Female athletes are at a much higher risk of ACL injury than their male counterparts. It has been suggested that female athletes are at up to six times greater risk of ACL injury compared to males playing the same sport at the same level, although more conservative estimates suggest females have about double the risk. The knee is at risk of injury in situations where the foot is fixed on the floor and bearing weight, while the body continues to move. For example, a typical mechanism of ACL injury is landing off balance from a jump and externally rotating the thigh and trunk while the knee is flexed, internally rotated, and loaded.

Rupture of the ACL causes knee instability in rotation and anterior translation and abduction laxity. Losing this major stabilizer of the knee places added stress on the secondary stabilizers, such as the joint capsule, collateral ligaments, and iliotibial band. About half of all ACL tears are surgically repaired.

Conservative (non-surgical) treatment options are available for those athletes who don't want to return to high-level sports, or those who are 'copers' and show no symptoms of instability after rupture of the ligament. In this case, the injury is treated with rehabilitation exercises and the use of knee bracing. The majority of athletes and other active individuals opt for surgical reconstruction of the ACL. The damaged ACL is typically replaced by a section of patellar or hamstrings tendon. This provides a stronger restraint than simply repairing the ruptured ligament. Following surgery, the athlete will spend six to eight weeks in a knee brace and undergo six to twelve months of rehabilitation before returning to play.

Further reading

Hewett, T.E. *et al.* (eds) (2007) *Understanding and Preventing Noncontact ACL Injuries*, Champaign, IL: Human Kinetics.

Ligaments

Ligaments are soft tissue structures which connect bone to bone at a joint. They are generally inelastic, and their major role is to prevent excessive joint motion. When the ligament is pulled tight by movement of the bones, it prevents further movement. In this way ligaments contribute to joint stability. Although they can't be stretched much, ligaments are flexible. They can be thought of as a short piece of string connecting two bones, which can move with the bones until it is pulled tight, when it resists further movement in that direction. Ligaments are composed mainly of collagen fibers, which are inelastic. Other components include water, fibroblast cells, ground substance, and elastin. Most ligaments contain only a very small amount of elastin, which is an elastic fiber. However, there is a spinal ligament with special elastic properties which contains twice as much elastin as collagen. This yellow-colored ligament is called the ligamentum flavum and it runs the length of the vertebral column. It plays an important role in spinal stability. This ligament is stretched when the trunk is flexed and recoils when the trunk extends from the flexed position. This elastic recoil assists with the extension movement of the trunk (*see* **thoracic region – ligaments**).

Excessive torque at a joint can rupture a ligament. Common examples of ligament rupture include rolling or spraining an ankle, when the foot inverts excessively and ligaments on the lateral side of the ankle are torn, and anterior cruciate ligament rupture (*see* **Hot Topic 4**). Since ligaments do not have a very good blood supply, healing can be slow and the ligament may take a long time to return to its original strength. Once a ligament injury has occurred, it is common to injure the same tissue again in the future.

See also **ankle and foot – ligaments; elbow and forearm – ligaments; head and neck – ligaments; hip – ligaments; knee – ligaments; lumbar spine and pelvis – ligaments; shoulder complex – ligaments; thoracic region – ligaments; wrist and hand – ligaments.**

Lumbar spine and pelvis

The pelvis is the link between the torso and the lower extremities and the lumbar spine is responsible for movement in this region. The pelvis is a rigid ring made up of several bones, some of which are fused and none of which allow more than a negligible amount of motion between their articulations. The five lumbar vertebrae allow a large range of extension in the lower back and a lesser range of flexion. As with all spinal motion, the movements between adjacent vertebrae are small, but the total for the five vertebrae becomes appreciable.

Since it is the link between the upper and lower body, this region is subject to large forces as movements are transferred between the upper and lower limbs. For example, in rowing forces generated at the feet against the foot plate must be transferred through the trunk to the hands on the oar to propel the oar through the water. This transfer of energy requires a strong and rigid trunk that will transfer and not absorb the power generated by the lower limbs. The lumbar spine is subjected to high loads during these activities. More importantly in terms of injury risk, it may also be in a weakened position because its can accommodate alignment faults elsewhere in the body to place the lower extremities where they need to be.

Further reading

Caldwell, J.S. *et al.* (2003) 'The effects of repetitive motion on lumbar flexion and erector spinae muscle activity in rowers', *Clinical Biomechanics*, 18: 704–11.

See also **core stability; lumbar spine and pelvis; lumbar spine and pelvis – bones; lumbar spine and pelvis – joints; lumbar spine and pelvis – ligaments; lumbar spine and pelvis – muscles.**

Lumbar spine and pelvis – bones

The pelvis is the junction between the trunk and the lower extremities. It supports the spine and rests on the lower limbs. The pelvis is strong and sturdy and is made up of four bones: the two hip bones, plus the sacrum and coccyx of the distal spine (Figure 8). The bones form a ring with a large aperture in the middle; in females this aperture is the birth canal. The hip bones themselves are made up of three fused bones, the ilium, ischium, and pubis. The lumbar spine sits immediately on top of the sacrum and comprises five individual vertebrae. There are several differences in the structure of the male and female pelvis. Most notably, the female pelvis has a wider and more rounded pubic arch.

The pelvis consists of several articulations, between the sacrum and the ilium, the sacrum and the coccyx, and between the pubic bones. However, only very limited movement occurs between the sacrum and the coccyx, at the sacrococcygeal joint, and between the two pubic bones at the pubic symphysis. The lumbar spine is the most mobile part of this region, primarily in extension and flexion.

The pelvic region is a site of overuse injuries. In particular, stress fractures of the pelvis occur in runners. The exact mechanism of these fractures is unclear. Why, for example, do some runners suffer stress fractures more distally in the lower extremity whereas, in other cases, forces are transmitted up through the lower extremity without injury to its tissues and cause a stress fracture in the pelvis? Stress fractures developed through running can occur in most of the bones of the lower extremity and the reasons why they manifest themselves in different places in different runners are the subject of ongoing research in sports biomechanics. Women are more susceptible to pelvic stress fractures than males, but the reasons for this are also unknown. The difference in the incidence of injury may be related to anatomical differences or other factors related to the sex of the individual. Sports biomechanics researchers use advanced techniques, such as on-line motion analysis (*see* **Hot Topic** 3), to investigate these relationships and have been studying the interrelationships between anatomical, physiological, and

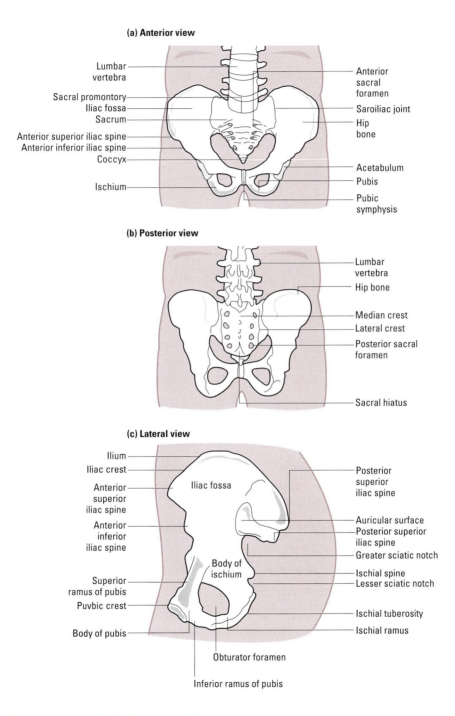

(a) Anterior view

Lumbar vertebra

Sacral promontory
Iliac fossa
Sacrum
Anterior superior iliac spine
Anterior inferior iliac spine
Coccyx

Ischium

Anterior sacral foramen

Saroiliac joint

Hip bone

Acetabulum
Pubis
Pubic symphysis

(b) Posterior view

Lumbar vertebra
Hip bone

Median crest
Lateral crest
Posterior sacral foramen

Sacral hiatus

(c) Lateral view

Ilium
Iliac crest
Anterior superior iliac spine
Anterior inferior iliac spine

Iliac fossa

Superior ramus of pubis
Puvbic crest

Body of pubis

Body of ischium

Posterior superior iliac spine

Auricular surface
Posterior superior iliac spine
Greater sciatic notch
Ischial spine
Lesser sciatic notch

Ischial tuberosity
Ischial ramus

Obturator foramen

Inferior ramus of pubis

Figure 8 Bones of the lumbar spine and pelvis

training factors and the occurrence of overuse injuries in running for more than twenty years.

Another group of athletes at risk of overuse injury in the lumbar and pelvic region are rowers, who commonly suffer from low back pain. Relationships between the dynamic position of the lumbar spine during rowing and low back pain have also been the subject of investigation by sports biomechanists and physical therapists in recent years (*see* **lumbar spine and pelvis – joints**).

See also **hip – joint; lumbar spine and pelvis; lumbar spine and pelvis – ligaments; lumbar spine and pelvis – muscles; vertebral structure.**

Lumbar spine and pelvis – joints

This region consists of the five lumbar vertebrae and the pelvis. The pelvis is made up of the two hip bones and the sacrum and coccyx of the spine. The pelvis itself is quite rigid and movements between its bones are minimal. However, the lumbar spine has a large extension motion and a more limited amount of flexion, both of which are the sum of relatively small movements at each intervertebral joint.

Acute injuries to the lower back can occur in many sports and are often related to the ballistic (explosive) movements involved. The lower back is particularly vulnerable when it is hyperextended, laterally flexed, and rotated and has a load applied to it. For example, in racket sports serving and playing shots while the spine is in this position can lead to muscular strains in the lower back. Weight lifting and weight training also places the back at risk of injury, particularly when heavy lifts are involved. Back injuries are often associated with poor technique or trying to lift too heavy a weight. Among the most common back injuries are spondylolysis (stress fracture of the vertebral arch), spondylosis (degeneration of an intervertebral disc), and spondylolisthesis (anterior misalignment of a vertebra resulting from a bilateral spondylolysis).

Rowers are another group of athletes at risk of overuse injury in this region of the back. Low back pain is common in rowers. Relationships between the dynamic position of the lumbar spine during the rowing movement and low back pain have been the subject of investigation by sports biomechanists and physical therapists in recent years. However, as with running overuse injuries, it remains unclear which factors are most important in this injury and, therefore, which individuals are most at risk of injury. Possible causes of injury include hip flexor tightness and lack of hip joint flexibility. During the rowing stroke, forward flexion of the trunk should be achieved by hip flexion with the pelvis held in a neutral position. However, a lack of flexibility in this region leads to increased posterior pelvic tilt and, consequently, the necessary forward flexion is achieved through the next available structure with sufficient range of motion – the lumbar spine. The following simple hamstring length test can be applied simply to rowers to determine whether they have sufficient hamstring flexibility to be able to achieve the forward position of the trunk from hip flexion alone. With the athlete lying on their back, with the pelvis neutral, raise the straight leg into as much hip flexion as possible without losing the neutral tilt of the pelvis. If the leg reaches a vertical position (90° hip flexion) the movement can be achieved. If the rower fails to reach this position, hamstring tightness is restricting their ability to achieve trunk forward lean using the correct and safest technique.

See also **lumbar spine and pelvis; lumbar spine and pelvis – bones; lumbar spine and pelvis – ligaments; lumbar spine and pelvis – muscles.**

Lumbar spine and pelvis – ligaments

The lumbar spine and pelvis support and transmit the weight of the upper body to the lower extremities. The pelvis has a limited amount of movement between its bones and is supported by strong ligaments. The sacroiliac joint has a very limited amount of movement and is supported by the strong posterior and interosseous sacroiliac ligaments, plus the thinner anterior sacroiliac ligament. The interosseous ligaments are the primary structures involved in the transfer of upper body weight to the pelvis and then to the lower extremities. Movement at the sacroiliac joint is further held in check by the strong sacrotuberous ligaments. These ligaments run from the sacrum to the ischial tuberosity of the pelvis and prevent superior rotation of the inferior end of the sacrum. The lumbosacral joint is supported by the iliolumbar ligaments which run from the transverse processes of the fifth lumbar vertebra to the iliac bones of the pelvis. There is also a joint between the sacrum and coccyx, although it does not contribute to weight transfer to the lower extremities. The sacrococcygeal joint is supported by anterior and posterior sacrococcygeal ligaments, which run longitudinally from the sacrum to the coccyx.

The lumbar spine is the distal end of the mobile portion of the vertebral column. The vertebral bodies are large and strong and the articular facets are oriented obliquely to prevent intervertebral rotation movements. The lumbar spine has a large flexion – extension range of motion and is supported by the common longitudinally running ligaments of the vertebral column (*see* **thoracic region – ligaments**). The strong and wide anterior longitudinal ligament runs the length of the vertebral column and is attached to the anterior surface of the vertebral bodies and intervertebral discs; it helps to prevent hyperextension of the vertebral column. The thinner and weaker posterior longitudinal ligament is attached to the posterior surface of the intervertebral discs and lies inside the vertebral canal. The posterior wall of the vertebral canal is formed by the ligamentum flavum, which connects adjacent vertebral arches at the laminae. The remaining ligaments connect the various processes of the vertebrae. The interspinous ligaments lie between adjacent spinous processes and weakly connect them. The strong supraspinous ligament connects the tips of the spinous processes and helps to prevent hyperflexion. There are also thin and weak intertransverse ligaments in the lumbar region which connect adjacent transverse processes.

See also **lumbar spine and pelvis; lumbar spine and pelvis – bones; lumbar spine and pelvis – joints; lumbar spine and pelvis – muscles.**

Lumbar spine and pelvis – muscles

The muscles of the pelvis can be divided broadly into those that flex the hip and those that extend the hip. It should be noted that the muscles of the thigh also contribute to movements at the hip (*see* **hip – muscles**). The muscles of the lumbar spine contribute to flexion and extension of the lower back, and also play a key role in postural support and stability. This region is commonly affected by overuse injury; improving postural alignment and **core stability** is the key to preventing such injuries.

The hip extensors on the posterior side of the pelvis are the muscles of the buttocks – gluteus maximus, medius, and minimus – which make up the bulk of this region, plus tensor fasciae latae and the six deep lateral rotators of the thigh: piriformis, the internal and external obturators, gemellus superior and inferior, and quadratus femoris. The action of gluteus maximus is to extend and externally rotate the hip. Through its insertion into the iliotibial band of the thigh gluteus maximus also stabilizes the knee in extension. The posterior part of the gluteus medius also contributes to these hip movements, but its anterior part flexes the hip and internally rotates it. Gluteus medius also abducts the thigh. The smaller gluteus minimus contributes to the flexion, internal rotation, and abduction of the thigh carried out by the anterior part of gluteus medius.

The lumbar spine region contains the posterior muscles of the abdomen: psoas major and minor, iliacus, and quadratus lumborum. These muscles are responsible for posture, extending the lumbar spine and flexing it laterally. Spine extension occurs when the muscles on both sides of the trunk contract; lateral flexion occurs when only the muscles on the side that the trunk is flexed towards contract. Psoas major is a flexor of the hip as well as contributing to forward and lateral flexion of the lumbar spine. Psoas minor flexes the pelvis and lumbar spine and iliacus flexes the hip. Quadratus lumborum contributes to anterior and lateral flexion of the lumbar spine.

The front of the lumbar spine and pelvic region is the distal part of the abdomen and contains the internal and external obliques, transverse abdominals, rectus abdominis, and the small pyramidalis. These muscles hold the abdominal organs in place, flex the trunk anteriorly and laterally, and rotate it about its long axis. The transverse abdominals are major postural muscles and have recently received a lot of attention as a result of the key role they play in stabilizing the spine during many sports movements, both to protect the spine and to enable power transfer between body segments (*see* **core stability**).

The lumbar spine and pelvis are often involved in overuse injuries in sport. Low back pain is a common complaint in elite athletes and recreational sports people alike. Although the immediate pain usually resolves with rest, like most overuse injuries, the problem will return unless the root cause is determined and rectified. For example, in those sports that require a large anterior pelvic tilt to be maintained for long periods, the muscles responsible for this movement, mainly psoas major on the front of the pelvis, can become chronically shortened and prevent normal pelvic tilt from being achieved in the normal standing posture. Examples of such sports are rowing and cycling. However, low back problems can also occur in runners, since they need to maintain correct trunk and upper body posture while supporting themselves alternately on opposite legs during the running stride. This problem builds up slowly over a long time and the subtle change in posture may not be detected until it becomes severe enough to cause low back problems. For the trunk and upper body to remain upright in a standing position, the lumbar spine must hyperextend into increased lumbar lordosis to counteract the increased anterior tilt of the pelvis. Although this compensation does enable the upper trunk to maintain its normal position with respect to the rest of the body, it overloads the lumbar spine and predisposes it to overuse injury and the onset of low back pain.

A lordotic posture can be recognized by the increased concavity of the lower back when viewed from the side. The pelvic tilt can be estimated by measuring the angle between the horizontal and a line between the posterior superior iliac spines and the anterior superior iliac spines of the pelvis in the sagittal plane (*see* **planes and axes of movement**). In a normal standing posture with the pelvis held in a neutral position by the surrounding musculature, this measure of anterior pelvic tilt will be approximately 10°. With increased anterior tilt as described above, this value will increase with greater inclination of the pelvis. Once this root cause of the problem is recognized, remedial measures can be put in place to lengthen the hip flexor muscles of the pelvis and retrain the individual to recognize and maintain a neutral alignment of the pelvis and strengthen the associated postural muscles appropriately.

The gluteal muscles on the rear of the pelvis are well developed in sprint athletes such as track sprint runners and track cyclists. In these sports, the hip needs to be actively extended during every cycle of the running stride or pedal stroke. In sprint runners, these muscles are actively contracted to bring the body forwards over the standing leg during the stance phase of the running cycle. This is a closed chain movement of hip extension, with the lower extremity in fixed contact with the ground and the body moving forward over it. Similarly in cycling, approximately half of the circular motion of the pedal stroke involves hip extension.

Strengthening muscles in this region takes several different forms. The large gluteal muscles can be developed effectively by weight training exercises of various types. Single joint exercises that isolate hip extension can be used, but compound exercises that involve all of the joints of the lower extremity might reflect more appropriately how the muscles are required to perform during sports activity. For example, in sports such as cycling and rowing, hip extension and knee extension occur simultaneously. This action is replicated during weight training by various squatting exercises. The postural muscles of the lumbar spine are trained and developed by more subtle means, such as locating and then maintaining the correct pelvic orientation. Supplementary techniques such as yoga and pilates are effective for this kind of strengthening.

See also core stability; hip; hip – joint; hip – muscles; lumbar spine and pelvis; lumbar spine and pelvis – bones; lumbar spine and pelvis – joints; lumbar spine and pelvis – ligaments.

Muscle

Muscles are the contractile tissues of the body. They can move body parts or alter the shape of the internal organs. Muscle cells are specialized to enable them to contract (*see* **skeletal muscle structure**). The individual cells are long and narrow and are referred to as muscle fibers. There are three types of muscle in the body, each with its own specialized activity. Skeletal muscle moves the bones at the joints, is under voluntary control via the somatic nervous system, and can be activated at will. This type of muscle is most important in functional anatomy and is covered in detail in its own section. The other two types of muscles are involuntary, meaning that they are controlled by the autonomic nervous system and cannot be activated at will. Cardiac muscle is found in the walls of the heart and the great vessels. Smooth muscle is found in the walls of most blood vessels and hollow organs such as the intestine. Cardiac muscle forms the myocardium, the muscular wall of the heart. It is also found in the walls of the aorta, pulmonary vein, and superior vena cava. Contractions of the cardiac muscle make the heart beat. Heart rate is controlled by the autonomic nervous system via specialized pacemaker cells. Cardiac muscle does not fatigue and contracts and relaxes continuously day and night for many years. Smooth muscle is found in the walls of most blood vessels, parts of the digestive tract, hair follicles, and in the eye. This type of involuntary muscle can remain partially contracted for long periods of time. For example, smooth muscle controls the thickness of the lens of the eye by squeezing it, enabling the eye to focus at different distances.

See also **ankle and foot – muscles; elbow and forearm – muscles; head and neck – muscles; hip – muscles; knee – muscles; lumbar spine and pelvis – muscles; muscle classification; muscle contraction – types; shoulder complex – muscles; skeletal muscle function; skeletal muscle structure; thoracic region – muscles; wrist and hand – muscles.**

Muscle classification

Muscles are organized into groups within body segments. These groups are separated by fascia (fibrous connective tissue) into individual compartments. For example, in the upper extremity there are three arm groups: the shoulder girdle, posterior arm, and anterior arm. Similarly, in the lower extremity there are anterior, medial, and posterior thigh compartments. Muscle names are derived from characteristics of where the muscle is found and what it does. Naming conventions include references to the location, shape, relative size, direction of fibers, number of origins, location of attachments, and the action of the muscle. They are often relative terms, comparing one muscle to another within the same segment. Understanding the classification of a muscle described by its name reveals important information about its location, structure, and function.

Muscles may be named according to their location and the body part they are associated with. Internal and external refers to being deeper or more superficial, for example, internal and external obliques on the trunk (*see* **trunk – muscles**). Anterior and posterior describes the muscle's position relative to a bone, such as tibialis anterior and posterior in the leg (*see* **ankle and foot – muscles**). Muscle names may explicitly include the names of body parts, such as the intercostal muscles between the ribs (costa = rib: *see* **thoracic region – muscles**) or the arm muscle brachialis (brachium = arm: *see* **elbow – muscles**). The overall shape of the muscle may be incorporated into the name: deltoid is triangular in shape (the symbol for the Greek letter delta is a triangle: *see* **shoulder complex – muscles**). Relative size is often used in naming muscles within a group. The gluteals are a good example, named from largest to smallest as gluteus maximus, medius, and minimus (*see* **lumbar spine and pelvis – muscles**). Pairs of muscles which are similar, with one being longer than the other (including the length of its tendon) are named as longus and brevis (long and short): for example, peroneus longus and brevis in the lower extremity (*see* **ankle and foot – muscles**). The direction in which the fibers of the muscle run can also be incorporated into the name. There are several good examples in the abdomen. The fibers of rectus abdominis are parallel to the midline of the body (*see* **lumbar spine and pelvis – muscles**). Transversus abdominis has fibers running perpendicular to the midline, horizontally around the abdomen. The fibers of the oblique muscles are at an oblique angle to the midline, running diagonally across the abdomen.

The number of origins, or heads, may be incorporated into the name as 'ceps'. Biceps brachii, triceps brachii, and quadriceps femoris have two, three, and fours heads respectively. Muscles may be named by the location of their origin and attachment, with the origin being named first, for example, brachioradialis originates on the arm (brachium) and inserts onto the radius. The action of the muscle may be incorporated into its name as flexor, extensor, adductor, or abductor. Adductor longus adducts the thigh at the hip (*see* **hip – muscles**). Muscle names may become quite long if they include a combination of these different classifications: extensor carpi radialis longus is a long wrist (carpi) extensor on the radial side of the forearm (*see* **wrist and hand – muscles**). This name incorporates the action, joint, location, and relative size of the muscle.

See also **head and neck – muscles; hip – muscles; knee – muscles; muscle; muscle contraction – types; skeletal muscle function; skeletal muscle structure.**

Muscle contraction – types

There are several different types of muscle contraction, which result in different movement patterns at the joint that the muscle crosses. In a concentric contraction, the muscle shortens as it is being stimulated. The direction of movement at the joint is in the same direction as the muscle torque being generated. A concentric contraction is what is typically thought of when one refers to 'flexing' a muscle; for example, concentric contraction of the biceps brachii (located anteriorly on the arm) results in elbow flexion, such as during a curl exercise holding a weight in the hand. Eccentric contraction is the opposite of concentric contraction. In this case, the muscle lengthens while being stimulated and the joint movement is in the opposite direction to the torque generated. Typically, eccentric contraction counteracts the action of gravity on the joint and slows down joint movement. Using the example of the biceps at the elbow again, the elbow joint will move from flexion into extension with eccentric contraction of the biceps. The action of gravity would naturally pull the weight downwards, moving the elbow into extension from the flexed position. The eccentric contraction of biceps counteracts gravity and allows the weight to be lowered slowly to the extended position of the elbow.

A third type of contraction is isometric, in which the muscle is being stimulated, but the joint does not move. In this case, there are two opposing torques which cancel each other out. The 'iso' part of the name means 'the same' and the 'metric' part refers to length. That is, the muscle stays the same length (compared to shortening in concentric and lengthening in eccentric contraction). In this case, there is typically a pair of muscles working against each other to keep the joint fixed in position. This pair of muscles is referred to as an agonist – antagonist pair. For example, to keep the elbow joint in a fixed position while holding a weight, such as flexed at 45°, the biceps and triceps would form an agonist – antagonist pair, since one is an elbow flexor and the other an elbow extensor. Isometric contraction is found in strength training and other activities when a joint needs to be fixed in position during the movement. In the arm curl example, the wrist is held in a fixed position to keep it in line with the forearm as the elbow flexes and extends. The wrist flexors and extensors are contracted isometrically to keep the wrist fixed.

There are two more types of muscle contraction which are special cases of concentric and eccentric contractions: isokinetic and isotonic. In an isokinetic muscle contraction, there is a constant speed of rotation of the joint. This type of movement is utilized in a rehabilitation setting, where an isokinetic dynamometer is used to restrict the joint motion to a fixed speed. An isotonic muscle contraction is one in which the amount of muscle tension or tone is kept constant. Since the effectiveness of a muscle in moving a joint may change depending on the angular position of the joint, the amount of muscle tension required to lift a weight may change at different stages of the movement. This is related to the line of action of the muscle across the joint and how close to the joint centre it passes. Strength training machines are often designed to create isotonic contractions during weight lifting exercises. For example, an arm curl machine is typically designed with a cam-shaped pulley for the cable to pass over between the joint and the weight stack, rather than a round pulley. The changing curvature of the cam pulley is designed to alter the resistance of the machine at different stages of the arm curl to keep the muscle tension constant, and the contraction isotonic. The rationale for this is that muscle strength will be evenly developed throughout the range of motion of the exercise. With traditional free weights, more muscle force is required at some stages of the movement than others, and the body develops in response to this.

See also **muscle; muscle classification; skeletal muscle function; skeletal muscle structure.**

Planes and axes of movement

There are three cardinal planes and three axes about which joint movement can occur. A plane is two-dimensional, like a page in a book or an image on a television screen. The only movement that can be clearly seen in a plane is one in which the body segments move within that plane. That is, they do not move towards or away from the plane, but within its two-dimensional space. In the following examples, assume that the person is stood in the **anatomical position**. The sagittal plane is the one seen when looking from the side. It divides the body into left and right halves (Figure 9). If you look at a person from the side, you can clearly see the movement of flexing and extending the knee. Knee flexion and extension occurs in the sagittal plane. The angle between the leg and thigh can be seen increasing and decreasing as the knee extends and flexes. However, abduction and adduction of the hip cannot be clearly seen in the sagittal plane. The changing angle between the thigh and trunk cannot be seen from the sagittal, or side, view. Hip abduction and adduction can be clearly seen if you look at the person from the front. This is the frontal, or coronal, plane; it divides the body into front and back halves. In addition to the sagittal and frontal planes, there is a horizontal plane, the transverse plane, which divides the body into top and bottom halves. Internal and external rotation movements of the body segments can be seen in this plane, such as internal and external rotation of the hip.

All joint movements can be considered to be rotations about an axis, like a door moving around the pins of its hinges, as one segment rotates about the other. There are three anatomical axes which are associated with the three cardinal planes. The flexion – extension movement that can be seen in the sagittal plane is rotation about a mediolateral axis. This axis lies parallel to the frontal plane and perpendicular to the sagittal plane. It runs from side to side across the joint and is sometimes referred to as the frontal axis. The abduction – adduction movement in the frontal plane is rotation about an anteroposterior axis. This axis lies parallel to the sagittal and perpendicular to the frontal plane and

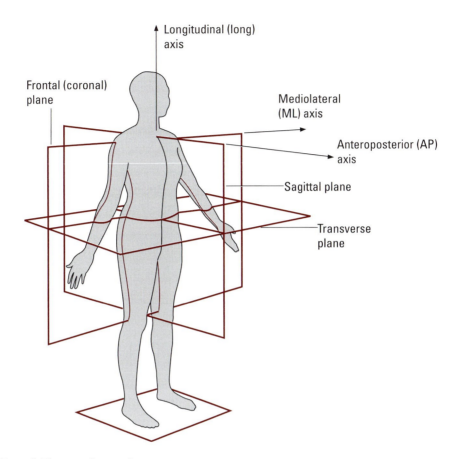

Longitudinal (long)
axis

Frontal (coronal)
plane

Mediolateral
(ML) axis

Anteroposterior (AP)
axis

Sagittal plane

Transverse
plane

Figure 9 Planes and axes of movement

is sometimes called the sagittal axis. Thirdly, internal and external rotations are about a vertical axis. This axis is parallel to both the frontal and sagittal planes and perpendicular to the transverse plane. It is also referred to as the longitudinal, or long, axis.

See also **anatomical position; anatomical terminology.**

Qualitative and quantitative analysis of movement

Movement can be described in one of two different ways: quantitatively or qualitatively. Quantitative analysis describes movement in numerical terms. For example, during walking the knee is usually flexed about 5° at footstrike and typically goes through an additional 18° of flexion as weight is transferred to the limb. The angles that joints move through are measured objectively using specialized instrumentation (*see* **Hot Topic 3**). The advantage of this type of quantitative analysis is that it is accurate and removes the subjective opinion of the observer from the analysis. The disadvantage is that that it requires specialized equipment to make the measurements. The equipment is expensive and requires a trained analyst to run it. On the other hand, qualitative analysis describes movement without measuring the exact angles that the joints move through. For example, during walking the knee is almost fully extended at footstrike and then flexes as weight is transferred to the limb. The description relies on the analyst's ability to recognize the critical features of the movement. The advantage of qualitative analysis is that it does not require any specialized equipment, and so is not restricted to a laboratory environment. The disadvantage is that it is subjective and based on the observations and opinions of the analyst. Qualitative analysis is also referred to as 'visual observation'.

Further reading

Knudson, D.V. and Morrison, C.S. (2002) *Qualitative Analysis of Human Movement*, 2nd edn, Champaign, IL: Human Kinetics.

Milner, C.E. (2007) 'Motion analysis using online systems', in C. Payton and R. Bartlett (eds) *Biomechanical Analysis of Movement in Sport and Exercise: The British Association of Sport and Exercise Sciences Guide*, Oxon: Routledge.

See also **gait analysis.**

Shoulder complex

The shoulder complex consists of the glenohumeral, acromioclavicular, and scapulothoracic joints. The glenohumeral joint is formed between the proximal end of the humerus and the glenoid fossa of the scapula (shoulder blade). It is a ball and socket joint (*see* **joints**) but, since the glenoid fossa is shallow, it relies on ligamentous and tendinous attachments to maintain its integrity and prevent dislocation. Owing to the structure of the joint, the shoulder is capable of movement in all three cardinal planes: flexion – extension, abduction – adduction, and internal – external rotation, plus the combined movement of circumduction (*see* **planes and axes of movement**). The range of motion of the glenohumeral joint is increased by movements at the scapulothoracic joint. Movement of the scapula on the back of the thoracic cage alters the position of the glenoid fossa and enables a greater range of motion to occur at the shoulder. This relationship is known as 'scapulohumeral rhythm'.

Owing to its structure, the shoulder is a flexible joint capable of maneuvering the arm and hand into a huge range of positions. However, this flexibility also puts the joint at risk of injury. Since the stability and integrity of the joint are maintained by soft tissue structures rather than bony anatomy, the soft tissues can be damaged if the load applied to them is too great. The shoulder is at risk of both traumatic and overuse injury. A typical traumatic injury is dislocation of the head of the humerus from the glenoid fossa of the scapula. This injury is relatively common in contact sports such as rugby, when contact with another player or the ground can result in a blow to the shoulder that is severe enough to force the humerus out of its shallow socket. Overuse injuries occur when a lower load is applied to the joint, but is applied repeatedly during the course of training and competition. Although such a load poses no threat to the integrity of the joint during an isolated episode of loading, the cumulative effects can cause sufficient microtrauma to damage the tissue faster than it can be repaired. An example of this type of injury is swimmer's shoulder, or subacromial impingement syndrome (*see* **shoulder complex – joints**).

See also **shoulder complex – bones; shoulder complex – joints; shoulder complex – ligaments; shoulder complex – muscles.**

Shoulder complex – bones

The shoulder is the most proximal joint of the upper extremity and has the greatest multiaxial range of motion of all the upper extremity joints. The glenohumeral joint is formed between the scapula (shoulder blade) and the humerus, the long bone in the upper arm that contributes to both the shoulder and the **elbow joint** (Figure 10). The glenohumeral joint is a ball and socket joint and, as such, makes the arm very mobile with respect to the torso. The joint has only a shallow socket in the glenoid fossa of the scapula for the humerus to sit in, but is protected against displacement by strong ligament and tendinous attachments. The shoulder complex comprises the glenohumeral joint plus the acromioclavicular joint, between the scapula and the lateral end of the clavicle (collarbone) and the scapulothoracic joint, between the subscapular fossa and the thoracic cage. The scapulothoracic joint is not a traditional joint, since bone does not articulate directly with bone (*see* **joint classification**). However, this structure makes a large contribution to the mobility of the shoulder complex.

The humerus is the longest bone of the upper limb and consists of a long diaphysis with a hemispherical head proximally at the shoulder joint. Distally the bone thickens out into the articular condyles that form the proximal part of the elbow joint. Overuse injuries of the upper extremity are less common than in the lower extremity, since the upper body is not subjected as frequently to high repetitions with high loading. However, overuse injuries of the upper extremity do occur in throwing and hitting sports and those that involve repetitive stereotyped movements; particularly at the glenohumeral joint, which relies heavily on soft tissue structures to maintain its integrity (*see* **shoulder complex**

– **joints**). Traumatic injuries to the bones of the shoulder are relatively common and typically result from a fall.

A common traumatic injury to the clavicle is fracture of the lateral or middle third of the bone. The most common mechanism of fracture is falling onto the outstretched arm and hand or directly onto the end of the shoulder. This particular injury may appear to be relatively minor, but it has the potential for serious complications because several important structures lie just below the bone: the top of the lung, the subclavian blood vessels, and a nervous structure known as the brachial plexus. To minimize the risk of this injury, learning how to fall properly in contact sports such as rugby and judo is essential and should be taught from the earliest stage of player development.

Another traumatic shoulder injury common to those contact sports is shoulder subluxation, or partial dislocation, more accurately described as acromioclavicular joint sprain. This injury tends to occur when the athlete falls directly onto the end of the shoulder. The severity of the injury depends on how much of the ligamentous structure spanning the joint is disrupted (*see* **shoulder complex – ligaments**).

See also **bone; bone classification; shoulder complex; shoulder complex – joint; shoulder complex – ligaments; shoulder complex – muscles**

Shoulder complex – joints

The shoulder complex has three individual joints, involving the scapula (shoulder blade), clavicle (collarbone), and the humerus. The glenohumeral joint is the most proximal joint of the upper extremity and has the greatest multiaxial range of motion of all the upper extremity joints. It is formed between the glenoid fossa of the scapula and the proximal end of the humerus. The shoulder joint is a ball and socket joint (*see* **joints**) and, as such, makes the arm very mobile in relation to the torso. The joint has only a shallow socket formed by the glenoid fossa of the scapula, against which the hemispherical head of the humerus sits; it is protected against dislocation by strong ligament

(a) Anterior view

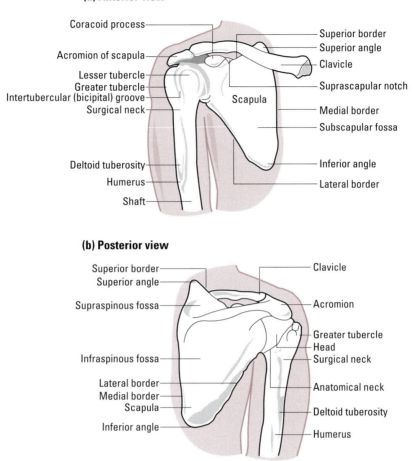

Coracoid process

Acromion of scapula

Lesser tubercle
Greater tubercle
Intertubercular (bicipital) groove
Surgical neck

Scapula

Superior border
Superior angle
Clavicle

Suprascapular notch

Medial border
Subscapular fossa

Deltoid tuberosity
Humerus
Shaft

Inferior angle
Lateral border

(b) Posterior view

Superior border
Superior angle

Supraspinous fossa

Clavicle

Acromion

Infraspinous fossa

Lateral border
Medial border
Scapula

Inferior angle

Greater tubercle
Head
Surgical neck

Anatomical neck

Deltoid tuberosity

Humerus

Figure 10 Bones of the right shoulder

and tendinous attachments. This arrangement enables the large ranges of motion at the joint but also puts it at greater risk of dislocation than the comparable lower extremity joint, the **hip joint**, which has a much deeper ball and socket and is, consequently, dislocated much less often. Movements possible at the glenohumeral joint are flexion, extension, abduction, adduction, internal rotation, external rotation, horizontal adduction, and horizontal abduction (*see* **planes and axes of movement**). Horizontal abduction and adduction are movements that occur only at the glenohumeral joint. The movements occur in the transverse plane, with horizontal adduction being movement towards the midline in this plane and horizontal abduction being movement away from the midline.

The two other joints of the shoulder complex are the acromioclavicular joint, between the lateral end of the clavicle and the scapula, and the scapulothoracic joint. The scapulothoracic joint is not a traditional joint in the sense of bone articulating directly with bone (*see* **joint classification**). Instead, the flattened scapula can glide over the posterior aspect of the thoracic cage. The scapula can elevate, depress, upwardly and downwardly rotate, retract (adduct) and protract (abduct) on the thorax. As a result of these movements, the position of the glenoid fossa of the scapula is altered and, as a consequence, the glenohumeral joint is moved. This arrangement enables a greater range of motion at the shoulder than would be possible by movement of the glenohumeral joint alone. The interaction between the scapulothoracic and glenohumeral joints is known as 'scapulohumeral rhythm'.

The shoulder is one of the most commonly injured sites in swimmers. Because their body weight is supported and the sport is a non-contact one, swimmers do not tend to suffer from traumatic injuries. However, overuse injuries are common, owing mainly to the stereotyped repetition of movements and large training loads of competitive swimmers. Because of the large range of shoulder motion required by the arm action in swimming, an injury known as 'swimmer's shoulder' or subacromial impingement syndrome may occur. This is inflammation of the tendon of supraspinatus, a shoulder muscle responsible for abduction of the arm, secondary to it being pinched under the acromion process of the scapula.

Dislocation of the glenohumeral joint is a common acute shoulder injury associated with contact team sports, such as rugby and American football. Shoulder dislocation is also common in individual contact sports such as judo and wrestling. The mechanism of injury is typically a fall onto an abducted and externally rotated arm. The other common acute injury at the shoulder is damage to the acromioclavicular ligaments, or a 'separated shoulder'. Falling on the outstretched arm or directly onto the point of the shoulder can results in damage to these ligaments, producing a noticeable step at the lateral end of the clavicle; the size of the step depends on the extent of disruption of the acromioclavicular ligaments and the adjacent coracoclavicular ligaments (*see* **shoulder complex – ligaments**). This cosmetic change may remain after the injury has healed but rarely affects athletic performance.

Further reading

Weldon, E.J. and Richardson, A.B. (2001) 'Upper extremity overuse injuries in swimming: A discussion of swimmer's shoulder', *Clinics in Sports Medicine*, 20: 423–38.

See also **shoulder complex; shoulder complex – bones; shoulder complex – muscles; thoracic region.**

Shoulder complex – ligaments

The synovial joints of the shoulder complex are the glenohumeral and acromioclavicular joints. The scapulothoracic articulation is not a traditional joint and does not have ligaments associated with it. The glenohumeral joint is the primary joint of the shoulder, between the trunk and upper extremity. This joint is a shallow ball and socket joint which relies on its soft tissue structures for stability and support.

The ligaments of the glenohumeral joint are thickenings of the joint capsule. They are the glenohumeral ligament and the coracohumeral ligament. The glenohumeral ligament is an anterior thickening of the joint capsule. It consists of superior, middle, and inferior parts. It is not particularly strong and is vulnerable to damage during traumatic injuries such as glenohumeral joint dislocation (*see* **shoulder complex – joints**). The coracohumeral ligament runs from the coracoid process of the scapula to the greater and lesser tubercles of the humerus. It is a superior thickening of the joint capsule. This strong ligament helps to support the weight of the upper limb which hangs from the glenoid fossa. Due to its lack of bony support and limited contribution from the glenohumeral ligament, the glenohumeral joint relies heavily on the muscles of the shoulder joint for support.

The acromioclavicular joint is also considered part of the shoulder girdle, since the acromion process is part of the scapula. Several ligaments connect the clavicle to the scapula. At this joint, the acromioclavicular ligament is a thickening of the joint capsule, equivalent to the glenohumeral ligament at the glenohumeral joint. In addition, coracoclavicular ligaments, between the coracoid process and the clavicle, assist in keeping the clavicle in place. These ligaments attach to the clavicle medial to the acromioclavicular joint and connect to the coracoid process inferiorly. There are two distinct coracoclavicular ligaments, the trapezoid and conoid, named according to their shape (trapezoidal and cone-shaped). The conoid is the more medial of the two. The important role of these ligaments becomes apparent after an acromioclavicular joint separation. This injury is a dislocation of the acromioclavicular joint which typically occurs as a result of a fall directly onto the shoulder. The severity of the injury is determined by the degree of separation of the clavicle from the acromion process. If only the acromioclavicular ligament is torn, there is no apparent separation of the joint because the coracoclavicular ligaments keep the clavicle in place. In a more severe injury the coracoclavicular ligaments are also torn, and the clavicle is now free to move superiorly and become separated from the acromion. In this case, the lateral end of the clavicle can be identified clearly under the skin as a bump on the superior aspect of the shoulder.

See also **shoulder complex; shoulder complex – bones; shoulder complex – joints; shoulder complex – ligaments; shoulder complex – muscles; thoracic region.**

Shoulder complex – muscles

The muscles of the shoulder are responsible for the multiaxial rotations that occur at the glenohumeral joint, as well as dynamic stabilization of the joint during activity. Muscular stabilization helps to prevent dislocation of the head of the humerus from its shallow socket in the glenoid fossa of the scapula. The muscles of the glenohumeral joint are deltoid, pectoralis major, coracobrachialis, latissimus dorsi, teres major, and the four rotator cuff muscles. The muscles of the rotator cuff are subscapularis, supraspinatus, infraspinatus, and teres minor. The muscles of the scapulothoracic joint are trapezius, rhomboid major and minor, levator scapula, pectoralis minor, and serratus anterior.

The most superficial muscle of the shoulder is the deltoid, which has anterior, middle, and posterior heads and gives the shoulder its characteristic rounded shape. As a whole, the deltoid abducts the arm. The anterior deltoid flexes and internally rotates the arm and the posterior deltoid extends and externally rotates the arm. Pectoralis major flexes and internally rotates the arm from its anatomical reference position. The muscle is a powerful horizontal adductor of the arm and an extensor of the arm from a vertical position. The latissimus dorsi extends, adducts, and internally rotates the arm. Teres major adducts and extends the arm and contributes to internal rotation. Coracobrachialis helps to flex and adduct the arm.

The glenohumeral joint relies heavily on its soft tissues to stabilize it because the glenoid fossa of the scapula provides only a shallow socket in which the head of the humerus sits (*see* **shoulder complex –**

joints). Stability of the joint is achieved passively by the ligaments that span the joint and functionally by the muscles surrounding the joint. Muscles are responsible for both joint rotation movements and drawing the bones together to strengthen the joint and maintain its integrity. The major role of the infraspinatus, supraspinatus, subscapularis, and teres minor muscles – the rotator cuff – is strengthening and stabilizing the shoulder joint by drawing the humerus into the glenoid fossa. The glenoid fossa is shallow and almost vertical in orientation, therefore the supraspinatus plays a major role in preventing downward dislocation of the humerus when carrying heavy weights in the hand. The infraspinatus and teres minor muscles also play a role in external rotation of the arm. Subscapularis is an internal rotator of the arm.

The muscles of the shoulder region can be strengthened primarily by various dumbbell exercises, which recruit different parts of the muscles depending on whether the dumbbell is raised to the front, side, or rear of the body. Dumbbell raises are single-joint exercises that isolate the movements of the shoulder. The shoulder muscles are also recruited in compound exercises that mainly involve the large chest or back muscles, such as bench press and rowing exercises respectively. In these exercises, which more closely mimic the likely role of the shoulder during activity, the shoulder muscles contribute to abduction, adduction, flexion, extension, horizontal abduction, and horizontal adduction at the shoulder, as well as providing stability of the shoulder joint and a strong link between the arms and the trunk. The dual role of the shoulder muscles in joint rotation and stability is well illustrated by the role of the shoulder in rowing. For a large part of the drive phase, the shoulder muscles are responsible for shoulder joint stability and the effective transfer of power from the lower body to the oar in the hands of the rower. However, at the end of the stroke, the shoulder muscles act concentrically in extending and then flexing the shoulder as the oar is removed from the water at the end of the stroke.

See also muscles; shoulder complex; shoulder complex – bones; shoulder complex – joints; shoulder complex – ligaments; thoracic region.

Skeletal muscle function

Skeletal muscle is voluntary muscle. Its primary function is to move the body at the joints. Skeletal muscle makes up about 40 per cent of body weight and there are more than 600 skeletal muscles in the body. Skeletal muscle has four major functions: movement, posture, joint stabilization, and heat generation. Skeletal muscle is attached to the bones of the skeleton via connective tissue (*see* **skeletal muscle structure**). The origin and insertion of a muscle are on different bones, with the muscle (or its tendon) crossing one or more joints. When the muscle contracts and shortens, it moves the bone at the joint the muscle crosses; coordinated movement of bones by muscles moves the whole body. Skeletal muscles also maintain body posture. Periodic contraction of the muscles enables the body to remain in a standing or sitting position. In addition to actively moving the joints, muscles are also involved in joint stabilization. A low level of muscle tone, in which the muscle is kept at a constant low level of contraction keeps tension on the muscle tendon and helps to stabilize the joint. This is especially important at joints like the shoulder and knee which do not get much stability from their bone structure. Finally, muscular contraction generates heat. Heat generation by muscles helps the body to maintain its normal temperature of 98.6°F (37°C).

See also **muscle; muscle classification; muscle contraction – types; skeletal muscle structure.**

Skeletal muscle structure

Skeletal muscle consists of muscle fibers (cells), connective tissue, blood vessels and nerves; it is surrounded by epimysium (sheath of connective tissue: epi = outside, myo = muscle). Within the muscle, bundles of muscle fibers are surrounded by perimysium (peri = around) and referred to as muscle fascicles. The individual muscle fiber is a single muscle cell and is surrounded by endomysium (endo = within). All of the connective tissue sheaths are continuous with the muscle tendons. Skeletal muscle can have either a direct or indirect attachment to bone. The most common indirect attachment is via a tendon, which is connective tissue that extends beyond the muscle. Tendons are rope-like cords which attach to bones at raised areas such as tubercles, tuberosities, processes, and spines (*see* **bony landmarks**). An aponeurosis is a flat sheet of connective tissue. A good example is the external oblique aponeurosis on the abdomen (*see* **lumbar spine and pelvis – muscles**). Muscles can also be attached directly to bones via short strands of connective tissue. These are referred to as direct or fleshy attachments.

Muscle fibers are highly specialized cells. They contain multiple cell nuclei because they develop from the fusion of many individual cells during embryonic development. The fibers are long cylindrical cells which are up to 100 microns in diameter (about 10 times greater than a typical cell) and tens of centimeters long. The microscopic structure of muscle fibers gives them a striped or striated appearance, hence the alternative name for skeletal muscle: striated muscle. Muscle fibers contain two types of muscle filament which slide over each other in contraction, thus shortening the muscle. The thick filaments consist of actin and ATPase (an enzyme that releases energy for the contraction). The thin filaments are actin. The filaments run in alternating parallel rows of thick and thin filaments along the length of the muscle fiber, with the ends of each row of fibers overlapping the ends of the next row. The pattern of striations on the muscle cell corresponds to the actin (I band) and myosin (A band) filament location, and the overlap between them. The H zone is the central part of the A band which is not overlapped with the actin filaments. The I band consists only of actin filaments. The M line is found in the middle of the H zone and runs perpendicular to the myosin filaments. The Z line is found running perpendicular to the rows of filaments in the middle of the actin filaments. The segment between adjacent Z lines is called a sarcomere; it is the basic unit of contraction. A myofibril is a row of many sarcomeres. The striations in adjacent myofibrils are aligned, thus the banding can be seen in the whole muscle fiber as stripes.

Muscle contraction is explained by the sliding filament theory. At each end of the thick filaments is a cross bridge (myosin head), which attaches to the adjacent thin filament at each end of the sarcomere. The cross bridge pulls the thin filament towards the centre of the sarcomere by swiveling inwards. It then releases the thin filament and returns to its original position, where it reattaches to the thin filament further along its length. The process repeats many times over during a contraction and the filaments slide over each other. The action of the cross bridge can be likened to pulling in a rope hand over hand.

See also **muscle; muscle classification; muscle contraction – types; skeletal muscle function.**

Thoracic region

The thoracic spine consists of twelve vertebrae and is less mobile than the flexible cervical spine above it (*see* **head and neck – bones**). There are twelve pairs of ribs in the thoracic cage. Each thoracic vertebra articulates with one or two pairs of ribs and the ribs are attached to the sternum anteriorly. As a result of participating in sports activities that require the thoracic spine to be held in a single position for long periods, the intervertebral joints can become stiff and the thoracic spine immobile. This can result in overload of the more flexible cervical spine, which becomes hypermobile to enable the head to maintain its position with respect to the rest of the body. In this situation, the spinal processes of the cervical vertebrae can become inflamed and painful to the touch.

See also **thoracic region – bones; thoracic region – joints; thoracic region – ligaments; thoracic region – muscles.**

Thoracic region – bones

The bones of the thoracic (chest) region are the thoracic vertebrae, sternum, clavicle, and ribs (Figure 11). The costal cartilages are also integral to the structure of this region. This region contains the heart and the lungs, around which the bones of the thorax form a protective cage. There are twelve thoracic vertebrae, each of which has two associated ribs. The ten superior pairs, seven pairs of true and three pairs of false ribs, are each attached to the sternum (breastbone) anteriorly by the costal cartilage. The first seven pairs of ribs articulate with the sternum directly via their own costal cartilage and are true ribs. The remaining three pairs of anteriorly secured ribs articulate only indirectly with the sternum via the costal cartilage of the rib above. The last two pairs are the floating (free) ribs, which do not have an anterior attachment and are attached only to the eleventh and twelfth lumbar vertebrae respectively. The sternum is divided into three parts. The manubrium is the most superior part and articulates with the first and second pairs of ribs and the clavicle. The body is the largest piece and articulates with the second to seventh pairs of ribs. The most distal part is the xiphoid process, which does not articulate with the ribs.

The basic structure of a rib consists of two ends and a body or shaft. The vertebral end is known as the head and articulates with the body of a thoracic vertebra. The rib tubercle, located anterior to the neck of the rib, has an articular facet that articulates with the vertebral transverse process. The anterior end of the rib articulates with the sternum via its own costal cartilage (true ribs), or indirectly via the costal cartilage of the rib above (false ribs). The floating ribs do not articulate with any bony structure anteriorly. The ribs increase in length from the first to the seventh; their length then decreases from the seventh to the twelfth. The body of the rib is grooved where the intercostal muscles of the thorax attach. Ribs are highly vascularized bones and consist mainly of cancellous bone inside a thin layer of compact **bone**. The first and second pairs of ribs are somewhat different in structure than the third to tenth pairs. The body of the first two pairs is flattened proximally to distally, whereas the remaining pairs are flattened medially to laterally. The angle (curve) of the first two pairs is also much sharper. The floating ribs also differ in structure from the typical ribs because they are much shorter, almost straight, and do not articulate with the transverse processes of the thoracic vertebrae.

Athletes who participate in contact sports are at risk of traumatic injury to the ribs. Although painful, these injuries are rarely serious and heal rapidly because the bone is highly vascularized. Overuse injuries can also occur in the thoracic region. This type of injury may occur when the thoracic region is under tension and forms a rigid link between the upper and lower body for the transfer of load. For example, rib stress fractures are relatively common in competitive rowers and are thought to be related to the forces transmitted through the body from the feet pushing against the foot stretcher of the boat to the oar in the hands.

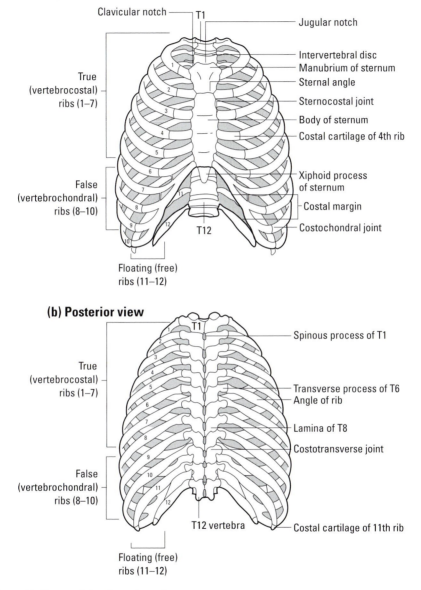

(a) Anterior view

Clavicular notch — T1

Jugular notch

Intervertebral disc
Manubrium of sternum
Sternal angle
Sternocostal joint
Body of sternum
Costal cartilage of 4th rib

True
(vertebrocostal)
ribs (1–7)

False
(vertebrochondral)
ribs (8–10)

Xiphoid process
of sternum
Costal margin
Costochondral joint

T12

Floating (free)
ribs (11–12)

(b) Posterior view

T1

Spinous process of T1

True
(vertebrocostal)
ribs (1–7)

Transverse process of T6
Angle of rib

Lamina of T8

Costotransverse joint

False
(vertebrochondral)
ribs (8–10)

T12 vertebra

Costal cartilage of 11th rib

Floating (free)
ribs (11–12)

Figure 11 Bones of the thoracic region

See also **bone; bone classification; core stability; thoracic region; thoracic region – joints; thoracic region – ligaments; thoracic region – muscles.**

Thoracic region – joints

The thoracic region consists of the thoracic spine, ribs, and sternum. The joints of this region are the sternoclavicular joint, the intervertebral joints, and the anterior and posterior articulations of the ribs. The thoracic spine is less mobile than the cervical spine, despite having more (12) vertebrae than the cervical spine (7). The sternoclavicular joint is formed between the sternal end of the clavicle and the clavicular notch of the manubrium of the sternum.

The intervertebral articulations of the thoracic spine are those between the vertebral bodies and those between the vertebral arches. These joints allow only small movements between adjacent vertebrae. However, when these small movements are summed across the whole of the thoracic spine, they add up to significant flexion and extension of the region as a whole. The articulations between the vertebral bodies are symphyses (*see* **joint classification**). The intervertebral discs are the main connection between adjacent vertebrae. These flexible discs of fibrous tissue and fibrocartilage act as shock absorbers for the spine as a whole and attenuate forces travelling up the body to protect the brain from exposure to excessive shock. The articulations between the inferior and superior articular processes on the vertebral arches are synovial gliding joints. The anterior and posterior longitudinal ligaments are associated with these articulations, as well as the intervertebral discs. The thoracic vertebral arches are connected by the following restraining ligaments: ligamentum flavum, supraspinous ligament, and interspinous ligament.

Joints found only in the thoracic region of the vertebral column are the costovertebral and costotransverse joints. These are the articulations between thoracic vertebrae and ribs. The costovertebral joint is between the vertebral body (*see* **vertebral structure**) and the head of the rib. The costotransverse joint is between the transverse process of the vertebra and the articular facet of the rib tubercle. Most ribs articulate with two adjacent vertebral bodies and the costotransverse joint is formed with the transverse process of the inferior vertebrae.

The spinal column can move in flexion, extension, lateral flexion, axial rotation, and circumduction. Overall, the largest movement is flexion, followed by extension, lateral flexion, and rotation. Only a little circumduction is possible in the spine. These movements are reduced in the thoracic region compared to the cervical region to prevent them interfering with breathing. The most significant movement in the thoracic region is axial rotation (*see* **planes and axes of movement**). Flexion and extension are reduced by the articular processes of the vertebrae being directed anteriorly and posteriorly; lateral flexion is restricted by the presence of the ribs and sternum.

The cartilaginous joints between the anterior part of the ribs and the sternum are a weak point that is subject to dislocation injury. In sporting activities in which the trunk acts as a rigid link between the upper and lower body for the transfer of power, the joints of the thoracic region are under considerable tension. This occurs in rowing, and rowers are susceptible to instances of the tip of a rib being dislocated or 'popping out' of its anterior articulation with the sternum. A similar injury can occur with the simple act of coughing. Again, the tension generated in the torso results in one of the ribs becoming dislocated anteriorly. This injury is particularly painful while breathing in and is easily localized to the dislocated rib. Typical treatment for this injury is physiotherapy that mobilizes this region and actively pushes the displaced rib back into the correct position. Relocation of the rib provides an immediate reduction in pain and is key to having a thorax that is stable under tension.

See also **thoracic region; thoracic region – bones; thoracic region – ligaments; thoracic region – muscles.**

Thoracic region – ligaments

The thoracic region contains many joints, and each has several ligaments associated with it. In the thoracic spine are the intervertebral, costovertebral, and costotransverse joints. The vertebral column has several ligaments which run its whole length, connecting all of the vertebrae together, either as one continuous long ligament or a series of shorter ligaments found between each adjacent pair of vertebrae. From anterior to posterior these are the anterior longitudinal ligament, the posterior longitudinal ligament, the ligamentum flavum, the interspinous ligaments, and the supraspinous ligament.

The anterior longitudinal ligament is wide and strong. It runs along the anterior side of the vertebral bodies and attaches to both the vertebrae and intervertebral discs. It helps to prevent hyperextension of the back. The posterior longitudinal ligament is narrower and weaker than the anterior ligament. It runs along the posterior side of the vertebral bodies, inside the vertebral canal (*see* **vertebral structure**). This ligament attaches only to the intervertebral discs and its role is to help prevent hyperflexion of the spine. The ligamentum flava are a series of ligaments which join the laminae of adjacent vertebral arches together, making up the posterior wall of the vertebral canal. They derive their name from their unusual yellow color ('flavum' in Latin), which is due to their high elastin content. Ligaments are usually inextensible cords, but the ligamentum flavum is more like an elastic band. It stretches when the trunk flexes, which helps to prevent rapid flexion that might result in injury to the intervertebral discs. It then recoils as the trunk extends and assists with this movement. The interspinous ligaments link the bodies of adjacent spinous processes throughout the vertebral column, and are relatively weak. The supraspinous ligament connects the tips of the spinous processes and is much stronger, helping to prevent hyperflexion of the back. Additional, smaller ligaments include the intertransverse ligaments, which link adjacent transverse processes. These are stronger in the thoracic region than elsewhere in the vertebral column.

There are two types of joint between the ribs and the vertebrae in the thoracic region: the costovertebral and costotransverse joints. The costovertebral joint is between the head of the rib and the vertebral body. The radiate ligament crosses this joint. The ligament is so named because it fans out from the head of the rib to its insertions on the vertebral body. The costotransverse joint is between the tubercle of the rib and the transverse process of the vertebra. There are lateral and superior costotransverse ligaments at this joint. The lateral costotransverse ligament passes from the rib tubercle to the transverse process it articulates with. The superior costotransverse ligament passes from the superior border of the rib to the transverse process of the vertebra above.

The sternoclavicular joint, between the sternum of the thoracic cage and the clavicle, has several ligaments associated with it. There are anterior and posterior sternoclavicular ligaments which pass directly across the joint. In addition, there is an interclavicular ligament which passes between the right and left clavicles, across the suprasternal notch. There is also a costoclavicular ligament lateral to the joint. This ligament passes from the first rib to the clavicle and assists in keeping the medial end of the clavicle in place.

See also **shoulder complex – joints; thoracic region; thoracic region – bones; thoracic region – joints; thoracic region – muscles.**

Thoracic region – muscles

The muscles of the thorax often play dual roles, generating movement in the thorax and shoulder through concentric contraction (*see* **muscle contraction – types**) and stabilizing the upper body through eccentric or isometric contraction. The muscles of this region are at risk of traumatic injury, in the form of muscle strains and tears sustained during ballistic activities, and overuse injury that often results from imbalances in muscular development.

The muscles that connect the upper limb to the vertebral column are trapezius, latissimus dorsi, the major and minor rhomboids, and the levator scapulae (*see* **shoulder complex – muscles**). The trapezius also contributes to neck extension movements (*see* **head and neck – muscles**). The muscles that connect the upper limb to the anterior and lateral thorax are pectoralis major and minor, and serratus anterior.

The muscles of the thorax itself are the internal and external intercostals, subcostals, transverse thoracis, levatores costarum, inferior and superior serratus posterior, and the diaphragm. The eleven intercostal muscles lie between the ribs and draw adjacent ribs together. When the first rib is braced by the scalene muscles that run between it and the cervical vertebrae, the external intercostals increase the volume of the thoracic cavity by raising the ribs on contraction. Conversely, when the last rib is braced by the quadratus lumborum muscle in the lumbar region, the internal intercostals decrease the volume of the thoracic cavity. Similarly, the action of transversus thoracis is to draw the anterior part of the ribs distally and decrease the volume of the thoracic cavity. The levatores costarum and superior serratus posterior raise the ribs and increase the thoracic volume. The inferior serratus posterior draws the distal ribs outwards and downwards, counteracting the inward pull of the diaphragm.

The diaphragm is a musculofibrous sheet that separates the thoracic cavity, containing the lungs and the heart, from the abdominal cavity. The diaphragm plays a key role in breathing because it changes the volume and pressure in the thoracic cavity as it moves. During inhalation, the diaphragm lowers and flattens, increasing the volume and decreasing the pressure within the thoracic cavity. Consequently, the ambient air pressure outside the body is higher than that within the thorax, and air is forced into the lungs. During exhalation, the opposite occurs and the decrease in volume and increase in pressure within the thorax force air out of the lungs.

The deep muscles of the back as a whole act as trunk extensors. This group includes the erector spinae, the splenius, semispinalis, multifidus, interspinales, and intertranservsarii. These deep spinal muscles are also involved in stabilizing the trunk, particularly multifidus, which works in conjunction with the transverse abdominals to stabilize the lumbar region (*see* **core stability**).

The thoracic region is subject to both traumatic and overuse injuries. Traumatic muscle strains and tears occur in sports, such as squash, which demand rapid movements of the torso and frequently place the spine in twisted and hyperextended positions.

Activities that involve one side of the body more than the other have the potential to create muscular imbalances that may lead to more serious bony misalignment problems if they are allowed to persist unchecked. For example, sweep oar rowing, in which the rower has only one oar, emphasizes twisting and leaning of the trunk towards the side that the oar is on. Since rowing is an activity that requires much strength and muscular development in the trunk, this can lead to the development of strength imbalances and asymmetries. Eventually, these muscular imbalances can lead to skeletal changes and introduce scoliosis into the spine of the rower, such that it is possible to determine which side the athlete rows on by looking at the inclination of the shoulders in the frontal plane. The rowing action encourages the shoulder nearest to the oar to be held lower than the outside shoulder to enable a longer stroke to be obtained. The best prevention against the development of these structural imbalances is to ensure that supplementary training, such as weight lifting, focuses on the symmetrical development of strength on both sides of the body. Similarly, flexibility programs should be designed to ensure that flexibility of the shoulders, trunk, and the lower extremities is symmetrical, and that any muscle shortening that develops as a result of the rowing technique is counteracting by actively working to stretch and lengthen the muscle groups involved.

There are many weight lifting exercises that will strengthen the muscles of the thoracic region; these can be divided into single joint isolation exercises and compound exercises. In general, compound exercises reflect the action of muscles during sports activities more closely, since it is quite unusual for an activity to involve movement only at a single joint. Examples of compound exercises for the muscles of the thorax include chest presses and back rows. Chest presses of all types develop the pectoralis major mainly and also parts of the deltoid and the triceps, which are involved in movement and stabilization of the upper extremity. Back rows develop the latissimus dorsi, plus the trapezius, rhomboids, and parts of the deltoid and the biceps brachii that are involved in stabilization of the scapula and movement of the arms during the exercise.

See also **muscle; thoracic region; thoracic region – bones; thoracic region – joints; thoracic region – ligaments; shoulder complex – muscles.**

Vertebral structure

There are 33 vertebrae in the human spine, divided into four regions. From the base of the skull down, these are the seven cervical vertebrae of the neck, twelve thoracic vertebrae of the upper and middle back, five lumbar vertebrae in the lower back, and the fused vertebrae of the pelvic region. There are five fused vertebrae in the sacrum and four in the coccyx. The vertebrae within a section are numbered in a superior to inferior direction.

The basic structure of the 24 movable vertebrae is similar (Figure 12). The main body of a vertebra is roughly cylindrical and oriented anteriorly, in front of the spinal cord. Immediately posterior to the body is a hole (vertebral foramen), through which the spinal cord passes down the entire length of the vertebral column. The bony structure surrounding the vertebral canal is known as the vertebral, or neural, arch. The parts of the arch that attach directly to the vertebral body are the two pedicles. The parts that surround the canal laterally and dorsally are the two laminae. Each vertebra has seven processes, four that articulate with adjacent vertebrae and three for muscular attachment. Each lamina has a superior and an inferior articular process, plus a transverse process for the attachment of muscles and ligaments. Each vertebra has a dorsally projecting spinous process.

The vertebrae of the different regions of the spine have slight variations from this basic structure. The cervical vertebrae are the smallest of the independently movable vertebrae and can be easily distinguished by the presence of an additional hole (transverse foramen) in each of the transverse processes. Several of them have interesting deviations from the basic structure described above. The first cervical vertebra is known as the atlas and has a ring-like structure without a defined vertebral body. The second cervical vertebra is called the axis because the atlas and the head rotate on it, around the dens of the axis. The dens is a superior projection on the anterior aspect of the axis. It provides a peg for the atlas to rotate around. The final, seventh, cervical vertebra has a long spinous process that can be palpated easily.

Thoracic vertebrae are the only ones with costal facets on the body and transverse processes for articulation with the ribs (*see* **thoracic region – joints**). Additionally, the orientation of the superior and inferior articular processes differs between the regions. In the thoracic region, the articular processes face posteriorly (superior processes) and anteriorly (inferior processes). This arrangement prevents flexion and extension from occurring in this region, but allows axial rotation. Lateral flexion is also possible, but is limited by the thoracic cage (*see* **thoracic region – bones**). In the lumbar vertebrae, the articular processes face posteromedially (superior) and anterolaterally (inferior). This provides rotational stability and allows flexion and extension to occur between adjacent vertebrae.

The size of the vertebrae increases down the spine, with the largest individual vertebrae being found in the lumbar spine. Overuse stress fractures can occur in the lumbar spine of cricket bowlers. This common injury, known as spondylolysis, is one of the few overuse injuries in sport that has been shown to have a statistically significant relationship to a particular technique. This injury is predominantly found in bowlers who use the mixed technique; this is a hybrid technique with aspects of both of the two traditional bowling techniques – front-on and side-on. The combination of a front-on lower body and a side-on upper body position during the delivery stride, when the forces being transmitted up the standing leg may be up to six times body weight, places the lumbar spine in a twisted, hyperextended, laterally flexed, and axially loaded position. Elucidation of this significant relationship has led to the mixed technique being actively discouraged in young bowlers.

Further reading

Bartlett, R.M. *et al.* (1996) 'The biomechanics of fast bowling in men's cricket: a review', *Journal of Sports Science*, 14: 403–24.

See also **axial skeleton; head and neck – bones; lumbar spine and pelvis – bones; thoracic region – bones.**

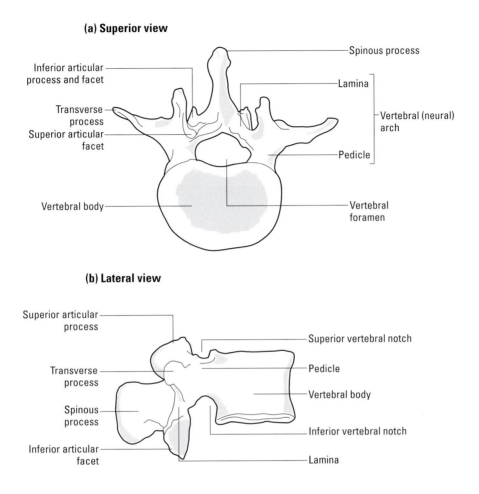

(a) Superior view

Spinous process

Inferior articular process and facet

Lamina

Vertebral (neural) arch

Transverse process

Superior articular facet

Pedicle

Vertebral body

Vertebral foramen

(b) Lateral view

Superior articular process

Superior vertebral notch

Transverse process

Pedicle

Vertebral body

Spinous process

Inferior vertebral notch

Inferior articular facet

Lamina

Figure 12   Structure of a typical vertebra

Wrist and hand

The wrist and hand complex has many joints, which provide flexibility and enable the hand to grasp and manipulate objects in the world around us. The many bones and joints in the hand enable it to perform multiple tasks during various activities. Each of the digits can operate independently, for example, when playing a musical instrument, or the hand can make use of the opposable thumb to encircle and hold various implements. Furthermore, owing to the flexibility of the shoulder joint (*see* **shoulder complex – joints**) and the **elbow and forearm joints,** the position of the hand relative to the body can be finely controlled.

When they are the main point of contact with equipment, the opponent, or the ground in sport activities, the wrist and hand are at risk of injury. Depending on the forces transmitted through the wrist and hand, and the frequency of force repetition, the athlete can be at risk of either traumatic or overuse injury. Traumatic injuries in this region include fracture of the scaphoid, the largest carpal bone, and the individual phalanges of the digits. Overuse injuries include cyclist's palsy, a neuropathy related to excessive pressure on the ulnar nerve at the wrist (*see* **wrist and hand – joints**).

See also **wrist and hand - bones; wrist and hand – joints; wrist and hand – ligaments; wrist and hand – muscles.**

Wrist and hand – bones

The wrist and hand contain many bones and joints, giving the region high flexibility. The hand is the major point of contact between the body and objects in the surrounding world; the flexibility of this region enables an individual to adapt easily to different holding and gripping requirements. The wrist and hand are also strong enough to support the entire body in sports such as gymnastics. The proximal bones of the wrist are the radius and ulna of the forearm (*see* **elbow and forearm – bones***)*. The eight carpal bones are the scaphoid, lunate, triquetral, pisiform, trapezium, trapezoid, capitate, and hamate. These bones are arranged in two rows; the first four are more proximal and the last four more distal. The bones of the hand are the five metacarpals and the fourteen phalanges of the digits – the thumb has two, whereas the fingers each have three (Figure 13).

The metacarpals of the hand are equivalent to the metatarsals of the foot (*see* **ankle and foot – bones**). They are long slender bones with a body and two articulating ends. The first metacarpal is that of the thumb and it articulates with the trapezium of the wrist. The second metacarpal articulates with the trapezium and the trapezoid as well as the third metacarpal. The third metacarpal articulates with the capitate of the wrist and the second and fourth metacarpals. The fourth metacarpal articulates with the third and fifth metacarpals, the capitate, and the hamate. The fifth metacarpal articulates with the fourth metacarpal and the hamate.

Although relatively uncommon, fracture of the scaphoid, the largest wrist bone, can occur as a result of a fall onto the outstretched hand. A fall of this nature can result in fracture of either the scaphoid or the radius, depending on the position of the wrist and hand at the moment of impact. Typically, if the wrist is fully extended, the scaphoid will fracture; lesser amounts of extension will likely result in fracture of the distal part of the radius. Acute fracture of the scaphoid may also occur as a result of striking an opponent in contact sports, such as rugby or American football, or in striking the ground or equipment with a hyperextended wrist in gymnastics. Although rare, this injury is potentially serious and may even be career-ending for the professional sports person as it has a high risk of complications.

See also **bone; bone classification; wrist and hand – joints; wrist and hand – ligaments; wrist and hand – muscles.**

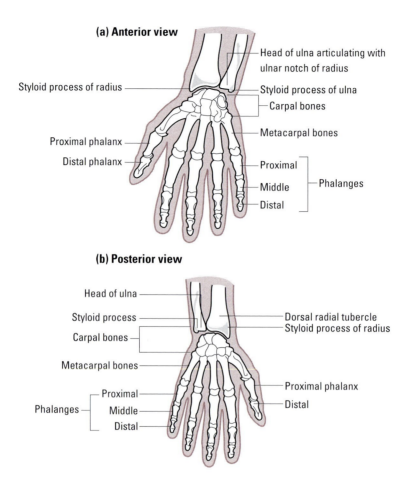

(a) Anterior view

Head of ulna articulating with ulnar notch of radius

Styloid process of radius

Styloid process of ulna

Carpal bones

Metacarpal bones

Proximal phalanx

Distal phalanx

Proximal

Middle

Distal

Phalanges

(b) Posterior view

Head of ulna

Styloid process

Carpal bones

Metacarpal bones

Dorsal radial tubercle

Styloid process of radius

Proximal phalanx

Distal

Phalanges

Proximal

Middle

Distal

Figure 13 Bones of the right hand and wrist

Wrist and hand – joints

The wrist and hand is a complex region containing many joints that provide flexibility and enable the hand to interact with its environment. This dexterity of the hand is essential because it provides direct interaction with the world around us and the objects in it. The major joint of this region is the radiocarpal (wrist) joint, the primary connection between the forearm and the hand. The bones of the carpal region have a little movement between them, mostly at the midcarpal joint between the proximal and distal rows of carpal bones. The intermetacarpal and carpometacarpal articulations give the palm of the hand its flexibility. The metacarpophalangeal joints – the knuckles – give the digits their independent movements and the interphalangeal joints enable the digits to flex and extend in grasping movements. Injuries of the wrist and hand can be both traumatic and overuse types.

The wrist is formed primarily between the distal end of the radius of the forearm and the carpal bones of the hand (radiocarpal joint) and indirectly with the ulna of the forearm (ulnocarpal joint); the ulna is separated from the carpal bones by an articular disc, although it is connected to them via ligaments. The carpal bones involved in the wrist joint are the scaphoid, lunate, and triquetral. These three bones together form a convex surface that articulates with the concave surface of the distal radius, forming a condyloid joint. The joint is supported by the palmar and dorsal radiocarpal and ulnar and radial collateral ligaments. The wrist is capable of flexion, extension, abduction, adduction, and circumduction movements. Extension is the largest movement occurring at the wrist, followed by flexion, then adduction, and abduction. Circumduction is achieved as a combination of these movements. No axial rotation is possible at the wrist; instead, this movement occurs through pronation and supination of the radius and ulna in the forearm (*see* **elbow and forearm – joints**).

The only carpometacarpal joint with any significant movement is that of the thumb – the first metacarpal. The movements permitted at this saddle joint are flexion and extension in the plane of the palm of the hand, abduction and adduction in a plane perpendicular to the palm of the hand, and opposition. The opposable thumb gives the hand its grasping ability by enabling the tip of the thumb to come into contact with the palmar surfaces of the fingers when they are slightly flexed. The ellipsoidal metacarpophalangeal joints, easily recognizable as the knuckles of the hand, also allow significant movement of the digits. This joint is capable of flexion and extension, abduction and adduction, and circumduction. Finally, the interphalangeal hinge joints of the fingers and thumb are capable of a large amount of flexion, enabling the hand to make a fist, and a little extension.

The wrist is prone to injury in a wide variety of sports. For example, the wrist is at risk of both traumatic and overuse injuries in gymnasts, as the upper limbs must often carry all of the body's weight in movements such as handsprings. Fractures and sprains of the wrist can occur when it is forced into hyperextension during a landing on the hands. Overuse injuries occur in gymnastics as a result of repetitive low-impact landings on the hands that do not load the joint sufficiently to cause an acute sprain or fracture, but instead cause microdamage that accumulates over time and eventually leads to injury as the damage accumulates faster than it can be repaired.

A common and potentially serious overuse injury that may occur in cyclists is 'cyclist's palsy', also known as ulnar neuropathy. This is a compression injury of the ulnar nerve at the wrist that causes tingling and numbness in the little finger and ring finger of the affected hand. If the injury is untreated and becomes more severe, it can lead to pain and weakness in the muscles of the hand and, eventually, coordination problems. If the injury is untreated the coordination problems may become permanent. The cause of this injury is cycling for long periods with the hands flexed and a large proportion of the body weight resting on them, resulting in the ulnar nerve being compressed. This position is most severe when the hands are on the dropped part of the handlebars. As with most overuse injuries, correction of the source of the problem is essential to prevent the injury from returning after recovery and rehabilitation. When trying to identify the root cause of the injury, consideration should be given to the time spent in the dropped position on the handlebars, the padding in the gloves and on the handlebars, and the position of the cyclist on the bike. If the bike is too long for the rider or the handlebars are too low, this will result in the weight being thrown forwards on to the hands, increasing the loading at the wrist. Changes in bike set-up may be essential to position the cyclist more favorably on the bike.

See also **wrist and hand; wrist and hand – bones; wrist and hand – ligaments; wrist and hand – muscles.**

Wrist and hand – ligaments

There are many bones in the wrist and hand. Thus there are many joints and many ligaments associated with these joints. Within the hand, the basic pattern of ligaments is repeated across the digits, with some differences occurring at the thumb. Furthermore, while the wrist contains eight individual carpal bones that articulate with each other, the distal forearm, and the proximal part of the hand, many of the ligaments restrain the wrist as a whole rather than individual components.

There are several ligaments that limit movement of the wrist, in addition to the joint capsule. The posterior radiocarpal ligament runs diagonally across the posterior aspect of the wrist from the distal end of the radius to the triquetral and hamate carpal bones on the ulnar side of the wrist. This ligament limits flexion of the wrist. The anterior radiocarpal ligament runs from the anterior aspect of the distal end of the radius to the scaphoid, lunate, and capitate bones of the wrist. This ligament limits extension of the wrist. The collateral ligaments of the wrist run along the sides of the joint to limit frontal plane motion. The ulnar collateral ligament, running from the styloid process of the ulna to the triquetral, limits abduction of the wrist. The radial collateral ligament, from the styloid process of the radius to the scaphoid bone, limits adduction of the wrist. Minimal movement occurs between the carpal bones themselves; they are held together by the anterior, posterior, and interosseous carpal ligaments. The interlocking structure of the carpal bones also provides support for the wrist, in addition to the support provided by these ligaments.

Anterior to the carpal bones, superficial to the flexor tendons which cross the wrist, is the transverse carpal ligament (also known as the flexor retinaculum). This ligament forms the anterior wall of the carpal tunnel (*see* **Hot Topic 5**) as it runs between the anterior prominences of the outer carpal bones on the radial and ulnar sides of the wrist.

Moving distally from the wrist to the fingertips, there are the following joints: carpometacarpal, intermetacarpal, metacarpophalangeal, and proximal and distal interphalangeal joints. Each joint has several ligaments associated with it. The carpometacarpal and intermetacarpal joints are supported by anterior, posterior, and interosseous ligaments. The metacarpophalangeal joint (knuckle) has a more complex arrangement of ligaments. Anteriorly, strong palmar ligaments run from the distal end of the metacarpal to the proximal end of the proximal phalanx. Medial and lateral collateral ligaments also pass from the metacarpal to the phalanx. Additionally, the second to fifth metacarpal heads are linked together by deep transverse metacarpal ligaments. The arrangement of palmar and collateral ligaments is repeated at the interphalangeal joints of the digits.

See also **wrist and hand; wrist and hand – bones; wrist and hand – joints; wrist and hand – muscles.**

Hot Topic 5: carpal tunnel syndrome in the workplace

Carpal tunnel syndrome is a common wrist injury among office workers and others who spend long periods of time typing or using a computer. It can occur as a result of any repetitive hand and finger movement that involves some application of force. It is also common amongst production line workers in meat and fish packing and car assembly. The vibrations associated with using power tools are another factor in the development of carpal tunnel syndrome. Musicians have a high incidence of this injury due to the repetitive nature of movements when playing an instrument. A modern risk factor for the development of carpal tunnel syndrome is playing computer games for extended periods of time.

The carpal tunnel is an enclosed space on the anterior aspect of the wrist; several flexor tendons plus the median nerve pass through it and into the hand. The tunnel is enclosed on three sides by the carpal bones of the wrist (*see* **wrist and hand – bones**). The tunnel is completed by the transverse carpal ligament, which makes the fourth wall of the tunnel. Problems arise when the median nerve is pinched or squeezed by the tendons in the tunnel. This can occur if one or more tendons become inflamed due to overuse injury. This is likely to occur if the hands are held fixed in extreme positions for long periods of time, or undergo repeated flexion or hyperextension movements, pressure at the base of the palm, or vibration. There is also a structural component to injury risk: if the cross-sectional area of the carpal tunnel is relatively small, it is more likely that tendon inflammation will squeeze the median nerve.

Symptoms of carpal tunnel syndrome include pain and tingling in the wrist and hand, especially at night. There may also be numbness in the thumb, index finger, and middle finger. In more extreme cases, the grip may be weak and it may be difficult to coordinate movement of the fingers. Treatment includes avoiding or minimizing the repetitive activity for a period of time. Patients often wear a wrist splint to maintain the wrist in a neutral position during daily activities and at night. Steroid injections are also an option to try and reduce the inflammation. As the tendons heal and the inflammation subsides, the nerve will no longer be pinched.

Long-term changes to the working environment that caused the injury should be made to prevent recurrence. For example, at the computer workstation the desk and chair height should be such that the wrist is held in a neutral position during typing and computer use. Keyboard trays which lower the keyboard to a level below the desk and wrist pads can assist with wrist positioning. In unresponsive or recurring cases, carpal tunnel release surgery is an option. In this surgery, the transverse carpal ligament is cut. Removing the restraint of the ligament as the fourth wall of the carpal tunnel effectively increases the cross-sectional area of the tunnel, providing more space for the tendons and nerve, reducing the likelihood of the nerve being pinched by the tendons. There is some risk of wrist weakness after the release of the transverse carpal ligament, although the surgery is successful in about 85 per cent of cases.

Wrist and hand – muscles

The wrist and hand complex contains many joints, providing an individual with the flexibility to interact successfully with the environment. This dexterity is essential because the hand is the means of direct interaction with objects in the external world. The major joint of this region is the radiocarpal joint, the connection between the forearm and the hand. Additional joints in the palm, knuckles, and the digits give the hand its ability to move and grasp items. The muscles of the wrist and extrinsic muscles of the hand are described elsewhere (*see* **elbow and forearm – muscles**), therefore, only the intrinsic muscles of the hand will be considered in detail here.

The muscles of the hand can be divided into three groups; those of the thumb (thenar muscles), the little finger (hypothenar muscles), and the palmar region between the metacarpals. The muscles of the thumb are abductor pollicis brevis, opponens pollicis, adductor pollicis, and flexor pollicis brevis, which variously abduct, adduct, and flex the thumb. Opponens pollicis also rotates the first metacarpal to bring the thumb in front of the palm facing the fingers, the opposed position that enables the hand to grip objects firmly between the thumb and fingers. The muscles of the little finger are the palmaris brevis, abductor digiti minimi, flexor digiti minimi brevis, and opponens digiti minimi. These muscles abduct and flex the little finger. The opponens digiti minimi also rotates the fifth metacarpal, so that the little finger faces the thumb; like the opposition of the thumb, this contributes to the ability of the hand to grasp effectively. The muscles of the palmar region are the lumbricals and the dorsal and palmar interossei, which flex the metacarpophalangeal joints (knuckles) and extend the interphalangeal joints of the fingers. The palmar interossei also adduct the fingers towards the middle finger and the dorsal interossei have the opposite function of abducting the fingers.

Hand injuries are relatively common in sports that require interaction with equipment, such as basketball. Many of these injuries are to bony structures, but traumatic injuries also include ligament ruptures in the digits; these injuries usually occur as a result of misjudging a catch. Hitting sports that involve the hand and wrist may put the wrist at risk of overuse injury from repeated movements under tension, particularly if the technique used is incorrect. For example, excessive tension and flexion of the wrist with the finger flexors activated can lead to carpal tunnel syndrome where the flexor tendons become inflamed through overuse. This is a potentially serious condition that may require surgical intervention (*see* **Hot Topic 5**). As with most overuse injuries, the root cause should be identified after recovery and rehabilitation from the injury to prevent recurrence once training is resumed. Errors in technique, or simply increasing training volume too quickly, are often causes of overuse injury, regardless of the specific sport involved.

See also **muscles; wrist and hand; wrist and hand – bones; wrist and hand – joints; wrist and hand – ligaments.**

Bibliography

There are many comprehensive anatomy textbooks available, represented by the entry for Standring, the classic reference text, below.

Bartlett, R.M., Stockill, N.P., Elliott, B.C. and Burnett A.F. (1996) 'The biomechanics of fast bowling in men's cricket: a review', *Journal of Sports Science*, 14: 403–24.

Bennell, K. and Brukner, P. (2005) 'Preventing and managing stress fractures in athletes', *Physical Therapy in Sport*, 6: 171–80.

Caldwell, J.S., McNair, P.J. and Williams, M. (2003) 'The effects of repetitive motion on lumbar flexion and erector spinae muscle activity in rowers', *Clinical Biomechanics*, 18: 704–11.

Collins, N., Bisset, L., McPoil, T. and Vicenzino, B. (2007) 'Foot orthoses in lower limb overuse conditions: a systematic review and meta-analysis', *Foot and Ankle International*, 28: 396–412.

Hewett, T.E., Shultz, S.L. and Griffin, L.Y. (eds) (2007) *Understanding and Preventing Noncontact ACL Injuries*, Champaign, IL: Human Kinetics.

Inman, V.T. (1976) *The Joints of the Ankle*, Baltimore, MD: Williams & Wilkins.

Knudson, D.V. and Morrison, C.S. (2002) *Qualitative Analysis of Human Movement*, 2nd edn, Champaign, IL: Human Kinetics.

Milner, C.E. (2007) 'Motion analysis using online systems', in C. Payton and R. Bartlett (eds) *Biomechanical Analysis of Movement in Sport and Exercise: The British Association of Sport and Exercise Sciences Guide*, Oxon: Routledge.

Nigg, B.M. and Herzog, W. (eds) (1999) *Biomechanics of the Musculo-skeletal System*, Chichester: Wiley.

Payton, C. and Bartlett, R. (eds) (2007) *Biomechanical Analysis of Movement in Sport and Exercise: The British Association of Sport and Exercise Sciences Guide*, Oxon: Routledge.

Perkins, R.H. and Davis, D. (2006) 'Musculoskeletal injuries in tennis', *Physical Medicine and Rehabilitation Clinics of North America*, 17: 609–31.

Perry, J. (1992) *Gait Analysis: Normal and Pathological Function*, Thorofare, NJ: SLACK Incorporated.

Sarrafian, S.K. (1993) *Anatomy of the Foot and Ankle: Descriptive, Topographic, Functional*, Philadelphia, PA: Lippincott Williams & Wilkins.

Standring, S. (ed.) (2005) *Gray's Anatomy: The Anatomical Basis of Clinical Practice*, New York, NY: Churchill Livingstone.

Warden, S.J., Gutschlag, F.R., Wajswelner, H. and Crossley, K.M. (2002) 'Aetiology of rib stress fracures in rowers', *Sports Medicine*, 32: 819–36.

Weldon, E.J. and Richardson, A.B. (2001) 'Upper extremity overuse injuries in swimming: A discussion of swimmer's shoulder', *Clinics in Sports Medicine*, 20: 423–38.

Whittle, M.W. (2001) *Gait Analysis: An Introduction*, Oxford: Butterworth Heinemann.

Willson, J.D., Dougherty, C.P., Ireland, M.L. and Davis, I.M. (2005) 'Core stability and its relationship to lower extremity function and injury', *Journal of the American Academy of Orthopaedic Surgeons*, 13: 316–25.

Index